DEVELOPMENT OF MEDICINE

ALISON HUGHES

CollinsEducational

This book is dedicated to my husband John and
sons Andrew and Malcolm.

Thanks are due to the following for their help and
encouragement: Val Squibb, Harold Butler, Vanessa
Benn and Malcolm Watson.

First published in 1988 by Holmes McDougall Ltd., Edinburgh

This edition 1992 by
HarperCollins*Publishers*
77–85 Fulham Palace Road
Hammersmith
London W6 8JB

Reprinted 1992

Illustrations by Harry Trowell and David Wilson.
Cover picture by permission of the British Museum.

ISBN 000 327111 0

Printed and bound in Great Britain by
Scotprint Ltd., Musselburgh

Contents

Introduction —
What is medicine?

Asking questions and getting answers

We want to find out what **medicine** is. You may think that medicine is a lot of different things.

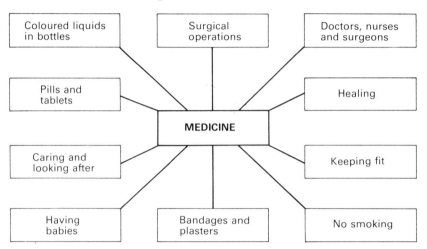

```
Coloured liquids          Surgical              Doctors, nurses
in bottles                operations            and surgeons

Pills and                                       Healing
tablets
                        MEDICINE
Caring and                                      Keeping fit
looking after

Having                    Bandages and          No smoking
babies                    plasters
```

? Make your own chart showing what things you think about when you hear the word **medicine**?

Look at **A**. Can you think of any other things to put on this chart? You may find that talking to a partner or a group of people might help you to think of other things.

Can you think of a sentence to tell us what medicine is? It might be something like the sentence shown in **B**.

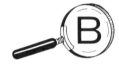

I try to help people who are ill to get better.

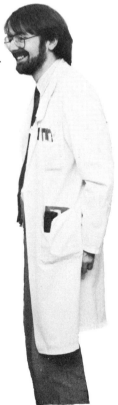

Look at **B**
? Who is this person?
? How do you know?
? Are there any **clues** in the picture?

The clues in **B** are called **evidence.** Evidence is important when we are trying to find out about something. The clues we look at are called source material. Reporters use evidence to write newspaper articles. Detectives look for evidence to find out what happened in a crime. Archaeologists dig up evidence from the past. Find out what reporters, detectives and archaeologists are. You might start by looking in a dictionary.

An **historian** has to be a mixture of all these things.

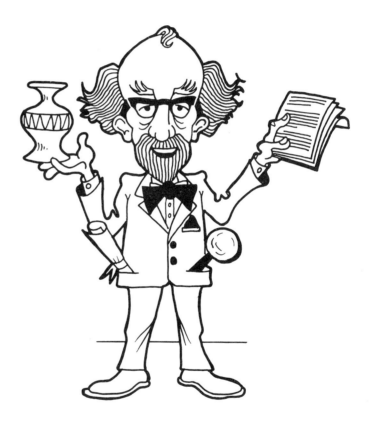

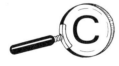

Look at **C**
? What questions might Professor Discover ask about medicine?

Look at **C**. It shows Professor Discover. He is an historian. He uses evidence from the past to find clues and answer questions. Watch out for his magnifying glass. It will show you sources of evidence.

We want to find out how medicine started. We want to find out how it changed. We want to discover how it became what it is today. We want to find out if it is likely to change again.

To find out all of these things we must travel backwards and forwards in time to find evidence and clues about medicine.

Medicine in the Stone Age

Key ideas

Evidence can be interpreted in many ways.

There seems to be a surprising amount of medical treatment.

There was a **dual approach** to medicine; magic and real treatments.

The Stone Age was a long time ago. It was 17,000 years ago. If the Stone Age was so many years ago how can we find out about it?

You might already know or guess some things about the Stone Age. We can find clues from a lot of different evidence.

The people in the Stone Age painted pictures on the walls of caves. Source A shows a picture from a cave in France.

Look at Source A
? Does Source A tell us anything about how people lived in the Stone Age?
? What animal is shown in the picture?
? What has happened to the large animal? How do you know?
? Why is the person falling over? Write any reasons you can think of why the person has a bird's head.

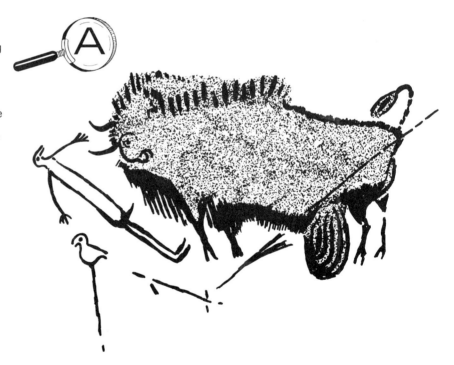

Source A tells us how people in the Stone Age found food. What name might we use to describe people who found their food this way? Did their way of life teach them anything about medicine? Clues: Injuries and cutting up animals for meat.

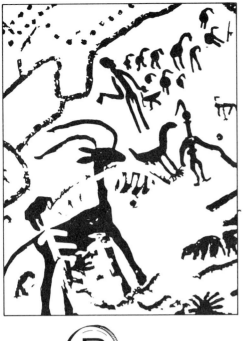

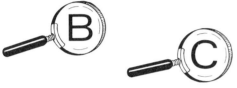

Look at Source B. It is another cave painting. It was discovered in Spain. The picture in Source B is very different from that in Source A. List all the differences you can see. Clues: Look at the people and animals. Look at the countryside. How is the life style of the people different? Do these pictures give us a good idea of Stone Age life? What parts of their lives have not been shown?

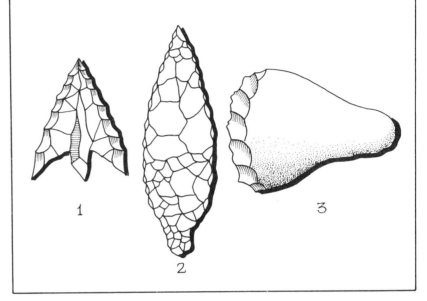

Look at Source C
? Can you guess what 1 and 2 are?
? How were they used?
? What animals might have been caught with them?
? What is 3? Why was it such an important tool for Stone Age communities?

Source C shows tools from the Stone Age. Tools like these have been found all over the world. They are another source of evidence about Stone Age people.

The tools and the paintings tell us that Stone Age people were **not** slow, hairy creatures who knew nothing. They were quite clever in some things. Their lives must have been very difficult. They had to face many dangers. What evidence have we seen of danger that they faced?

Dangers and survival

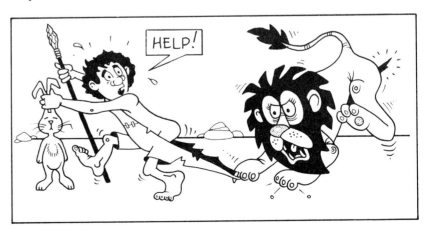

What sort of injuries might they have suffered in animal attacks? What would these injuries teach them about medicine?

7

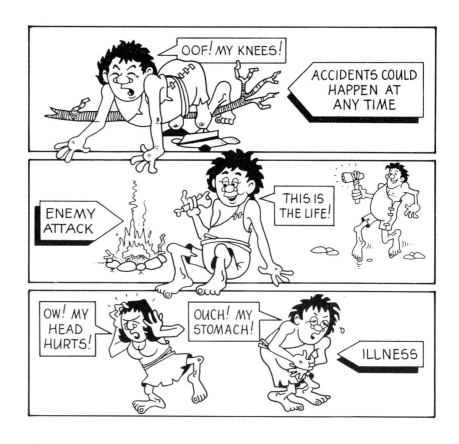

They managed to survive. If they hadn't, we would not be here now. What is survival? What things might they have relied on to help them survive?

Magic

How did they survive? There were no hospitals. There were no ambulances. There were no chemist shops. There weren't even any doctors or nurses. Or were there?

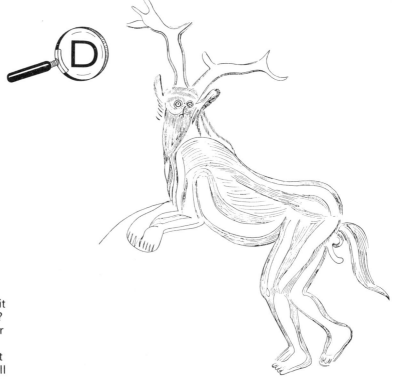

Look at Source D
? Who is this? Is it a person? Is it an animal? What do you think?
? If this is a person, why is he or she dressed in a deer skin? Could it be a disguise? Could it be a fancy-dress party? List all the reasons you can think of to explain this strange clothing.

Source D is called Antler Man. It appears in many cave paintings all over the world. It is usually in the middle of a circle of twelve people. Often other people are shown watching. You may have guessed that he was the medicine man of his tribe. He was a kind of priest. He was the leader of worship and celebration in the community. The other people believed he could do magic.

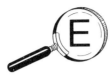

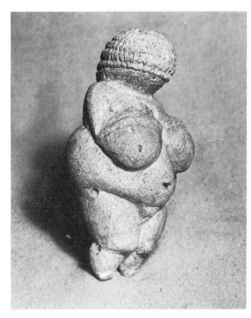

Look at Source E
? What sort of luck might these charms have brought?
? What sort of things would the medicine man ask the gods to give the tribe?

Source E shows a charm in the form of a large lady made by Stone Age people. Stone Age people often made charms for good luck. Bad luck and illness came from evil spirits. The Stone Age people believed life was organised by gods and goddesses. The medicine man did magic, so he could talk to the spirits. He was the go-between for his tribe and their gods. He was a very important person because of this.

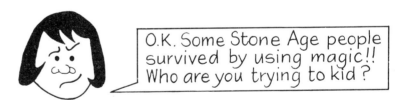

O.K. Some Stone Age people survived by using magic!! Who are you trying to kid?

They believed in magic but magic alone didn't ensure their survival. There is a lot of other evidence to consider.

Bones from the Stone Age have been found. They have been broken but someone has tried to mend them. The bones show new growth.

? How do you think Stone Age people tried to reset bones? You might think about all the materials that were handy, like wood, clay, mud and fat from the animals they hunted.

That's interesting. They were trying real cures, weren't they? Is there any other evidence to show the same thing?

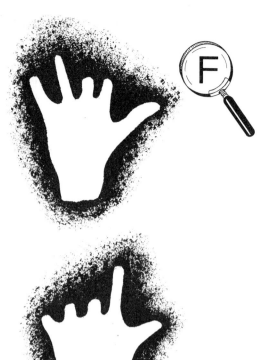

Look at Source F
? How do you think the hands were mutilated?

Surgical operations

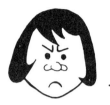

Yes. There is plenty of evidence. Some of it is very surprising.

Source F shows handprints from a cave wall in France. They show that at least two people from the same Stone Age community had lost some of their fingers.

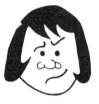

Ugh! How did that happen?

They could have lost their fingers in accidents. They could have chopped them off deliberately. American Indian women did this when someone they loved died. Stone Age people might have done the same thing. They might have amputated their fingers.

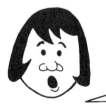

What does amputated mean?

It means cutting off part of the body. They lived in rough caves and huts. These would be dirty. Stone Age people had a lot of germs round them. Germs cause illness and disease. If these germs got into cuts or wounds they would cause soreness and swelling. This could kill them unless they cut off that bit of the body before infection spread.

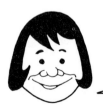

That sounds a very clever idea. I know that sometimes happens today. What other evidence is there?

This is the best evidence so far. Many skulls have been found all over the world. They are thousands of years old. They have holes in them.

Oh! I see. Their enemies bashed them on the head did they?

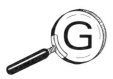

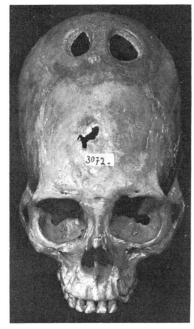

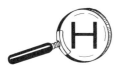

Look at Source G
? What do you notice about the holes?
? What tools do you think they might have used?

Sometimes, but some of the holes have been cut out very carefully. Source G shows a skull that has these holes. The holes have been made in the skull deliberately for some reason. This operation was called trephining. The operation was probably carried out to help people who suffered from headaches or mental illness. These were thought to be caused by evil spirits that had to be released. Some skulls show that the bone around the hole has regrown. Bone cannot grow if a patient is dead so some patients must have survived.

To prove that Stone Age people survived this serious operation, in 1961, in Peru, Dr Grama attempted the same operation on a young man with a brain tumour (growth). He used Stone Age tools. His patient survived.

What do you think would happen to the Stone Age patient during and after the operation?

Try to find out how operations in hospitals are carried out today. Talk to someone who has had an operation recently. Find out what happened to them.

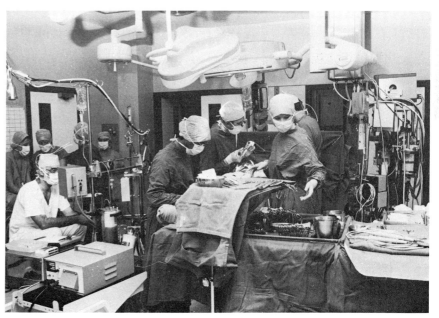

Look at Source H
? How is this operation different to that a Stone Age patient would have had?

Herbal medicine

Stone Age people were surrounded with plants and trees. Many of these would have provided them with food. They also used certain plants to try to cure illnesses. Who do you think would have gathered herbs and plants?

Pine needles give a fresh smell that can be used to help breathing. Many other leaves and plants were used to cure other illnesses. Stone Age people quickly learned the value of herbal medicine. They also knew what worked and what failed. How would they know what each plant could do? How might the herbs have been prepared? What tools might have been used in their preparation?

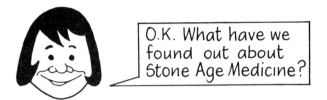

Stone Age people relied on magic to help them. Source I shows some more good luck charms made from pieces of bone.

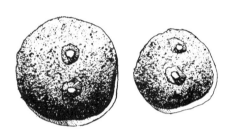

Look at Source I
? Where do you think the bone came from?
? How do you think they were used?

They also tried real cures. These sometimes worked. What real cures have we seen so far? Both magic and real cures might have worked for them. They used magic but they also had proper knowledge about some treatments for illness and injury. This was a **dual approach to medicine.**

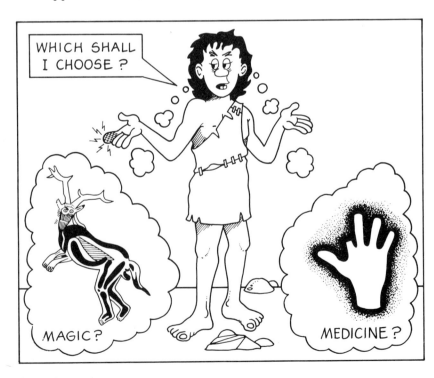

Stone Age ideas continue

There are still Aborigines living in Australia today. Some of them follow the same customs as their ancestors did for thousands of years. We can look at their customs and traditions as another source of evidence about early people and their medical treatments.

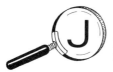

Source J shows an Aborigine medicine man. He was an important person in his community. He is massaging a patient with sweat from his own body.

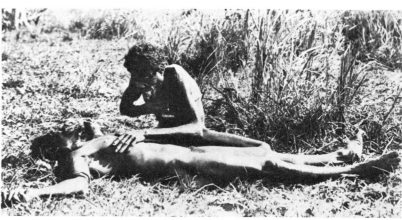

Look at Source J
? Why is the medicine man using his own sweat to massage the patient?
? When do you think he was alive:
(a) Stone Age
(b) 500 years ago
(c) Today?
? Why do you think he was alive in this time?

The Aborigines had many traditions about how the world was made. They had stories to explain how plants, people and animals were made. Some Aborigines today still have the same beliefs as their ancestors. Look at Source K. This is the Rainbow Serpent. Some Aborigines believe he is a good spirit. As he moved along he made rivers where he glided. Early Aborigines believed spirits like these were their ancestors. Some were good spirits. Some were bad. They left spirit children who could come alive in plants, animals or people. Can you think of any other stories that try to explain how the world was made?

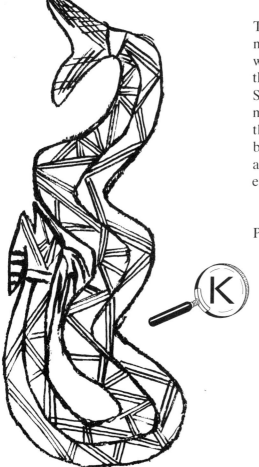

People were healthy as long as the good spirits stayed inside them.

The Aborigines were frightened of one thing. They believed that the spirit could escape through your mouth while you were asleep.

Look back to Source J. This shows the medicine man of the community. He sometimes used a pointing bone to try to recapture an escaped spirit. Who would ask the medicine man to recapture the spirit? Can you guess what happened to a person after the spirit left his body? Draw a cartoon to show this.

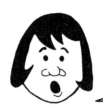

It seems to me that the Aborigine Medicine Man is doing what the Stone Age Medicine Man did. He is acting as a go-between. He can talk to the spirits and his community.

That's right. He can do magic. He is able to talk to the spirits and ask for their help. He can get good luck for the tribe. He can get rid of bad luck. He could protect the village against its enemies.

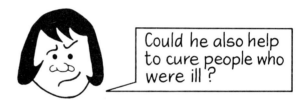

Could he also help to cure people who were ill?

Yes. He could use the magic of the pointing bone to cure illness. Source L shows a pointing bone.

Look at Source L
? What do you think the painting and carvings on it are supposed to be?
? How do you think it was carried?

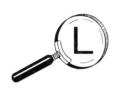

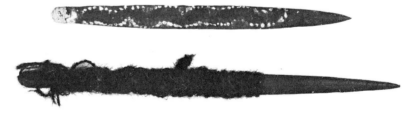

The pointing bone was made of bone, wood or stone. It was carved. Each community had their own special magic design. If it was pointed at an enemy it would capture his spirit. He would become weak.

If the pointing bone did not work, the medicine man would sell good luck charms. The best charms were made from parts of a human body. Why do you think these were the best charms?

Sometimes the Aborigines would take the hand of an enemy. They might wear it on a cord around their neck. Would this be a valuable possession? Why? Would Aborigines today still value this charm?

Medical treatment

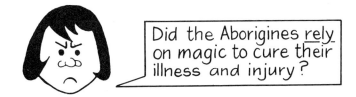

Did the Aborigines <u>rely</u> on magic to cure their illness and injury?

No. They tried cures that were not magic. Look back again to Source J. The medicine man massaged people who were ill. He rubbed them with sweat from his own armpits.

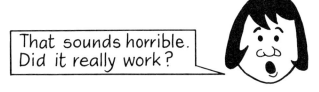

That sounds horrible. Did it really work?

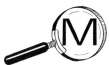

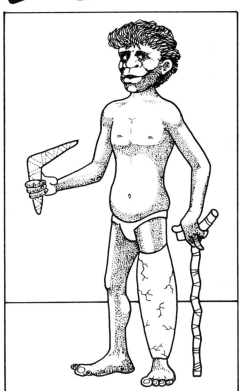

Look at Source M
? Would this be a good way of treating broken bones?
? Can you name todays equivalent of the Aborigine treatment?
? Do Stone Age people and Aborigines use the same medical treatment for anything?

We know that salty sweat massaged into the body revives people. Your heart pumps blood round your body. If the body is rubbed the heart sometimes works quicker. Blood travels round the veins and arteries more quickly.

The Aborigines enclosed broken limbs in mud and clay. This would set hard and stop movement.

They treated rheumatic pain with steam. This was made by putting damp grass on burning bark. Can you think of anything like this today?

They cleared their camps of human waste and rubbish. They carefully buried hair and nail clippings. This was because they didn't want their enemies to get hold of bits of their bodies. The enemies could use these to capture their spirits. This cleaning up had a good effect on their health. Why?

In Unit 1 we have seen that people who lived in the past tried some medical treatment. It was not perfect. It did not always work. But there was **some** progress. Some Aborigines still believe in the ideas of their ancestors. They also go to modern hospitals and receive scientific medical treatment. Does this still show a dual approach to medicine? Have their attitudes to medicine changed?

Ancient Egypt and other civilisations

Key ideas

Empathetic view of Egyptian life based on source material. Life and death and its effects on medicine.

Reconstruction of past events.

Understanding the ideas and treatments used in Ancient Egypt.

Who were the Ancient Egyptians?

Source A shows a Sphinx. It is in the desert in Egypt but it is close to the River Nile. In the background we can see pyramids. Pyramids are very big tombs. Dead kings were supposed to be entombed in them. The pyramids were built with big blocks of stone. Hundreds of slaves had to work to make the tombs.

Look at Source A
? What does the Great Sphinx look like? Try to draw a Sphinx in your book.
? Does the picture give you any idea of how big the Great Sphinx is?
? Why do you think the Great Sphinx was built?
? What do pyramids look like?
? Do the pyramids tell us anything about how the Ancient Egyptians lived and thought?

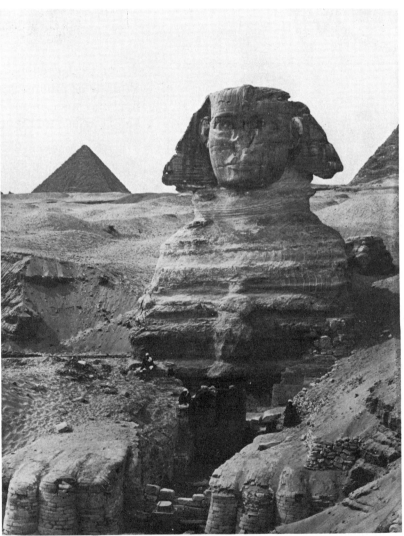

How do you think the big blocks of stone were moved? Do you think it was an easy job? Would the slaves have had any problems?

Imagine that you are a builder working for the Pharaoh in Ancient Egypt. How would **you** have organised the moving of large stone blocks and statues?

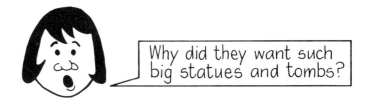

Why did they want such big statues and tombs?

The statues were for guarding the dead King. He needed help to keep evil away. Evil spirits could hurt him and stop him from going to the After-Life.

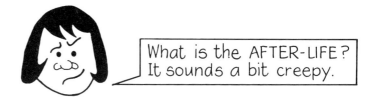

What is the AFTER-LIFE? It sounds a bit creepy.

Source B shows a dead King on his journey to the After-Life.

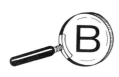

Look at Source B
? How is the King's body being transported?
? Who are the people accompanying him?
? What can you see with the body?

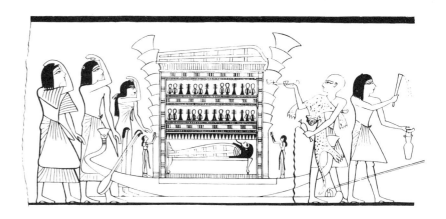

The Egyptians believed that when someone died they went to another life, which was better than their ordinary life. They would need all their belongings to make them even happier. When some Kings died their servants and pets were killed and buried with them. They would all go on to the After-Life.

Life and death

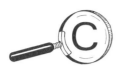

Source C shows a drawing of a very old grave in Egypt. It was uncovered by an archaeologist. There were 74 skeletons of men and women in it.

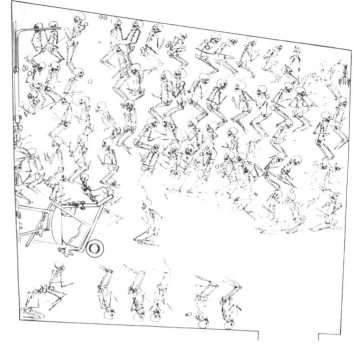

Look at Source C
? Do you think all of these people died at the same time? Why?
? What position are all of the skeletons lying in? Can you think of any reasons for this?
? What is your explanation of this grave pit?

They were probably the servants of a king. They might have been killed so that they could go with the king to the After-Life.

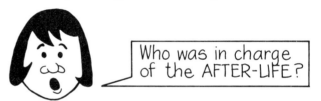

Who was in charge of the AFTER-LIFE?

The Egyptians had a lot of gods and goddesses. These looked after different things. Anubis guarded the gate to the After-Life. He had a jackal's head. He was supposed to weigh the soul of a dead person. By doing this he could see how good they were and if they deserved to go to the After-Life.

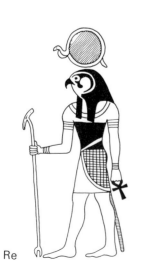

Re

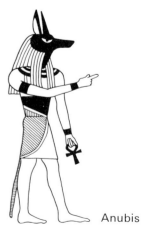

Anubis

Falcon-headed Re-Harakhte-Aten was the sun god. Winged goddesses protected people's bodies. There were a lot of other gods and goddesses. Sometimes they were called deities.

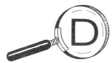

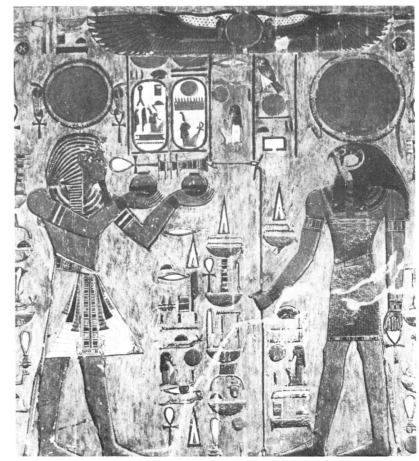

Look at Source D
? Who are the two people in the picture? What are they doing?
? Can you see the sun in the picture Why is it there?

The patterns on Source D are Egyptian writing. The writing is squiggles, patterns and drawings. Each line means a letter or part of a word. The writing is called hieroglyphics. One Egyptian King was called Ptolemy. Here is his name written in hieroglyphics.

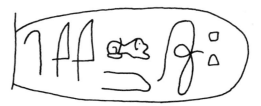

This name was carved on a very old stone. There were many other words on it. The words were in Greek as well as in Egyptian hieroglyphics. Because people understood the Greek words, hieroglyphics were made readable. The stone was called the Rosetta Stone. It is a valuable piece of evidence about Ancient Egypt because it tells us a lot about the people. Source E shows hieroglyphics on an Egyptian tomb.

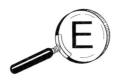

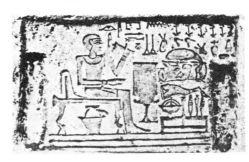

Hieroglyphics can be found in many places such as stones, pillars, tombs, coffins and papyrus documents. A lot of these papyri have been found by archaeologists. A famous papyrus was found at Luxor in Egypt by a man called Dr Ebers. It tells us a lot about medicine. There is a description of a human heart. There is a description of blood vessels. These are the little tubes that carry blood through your body. The papyrus tells us about herbs and medicines. It tells us that the Egyptians used to scratch the skin of ill people. If their skin started to bleed they might be cured.

From these written inscriptions we can tell that the Egyptians loved life. They hoped it would continue in much the same way after death. It was important to make sure that a dead person's spirit had a body to live in.

Why do you think the Egyptians had to deal with dead bodies quickly? If you were in an Egyptian household where someone had died, who would you send for to see to the body?

Mummification

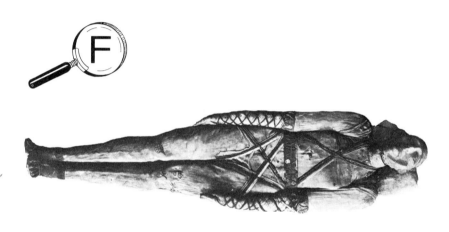

Look at Source F
? What clues does it give you about how the Egyptians made sure that spirits had a body to live in?
? What might the Ancient Egyptians have learned when they mummified a body?

This is a mummified body.

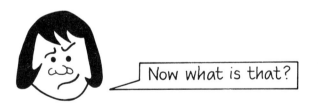

Now what is that?

It is what the Ancient Egyptians did to dead bodies, especially of important people. Look at Source G. It tells us how a mummy was made.

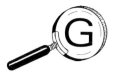

Source G. How to make a mummy

1　Cut the body from the left shoulder to the left hip.
2　Take out the insides. These will be needed again in the After-Life so place them in special canopic jars in preserving ointments.
3　Place the body on a mortuary table. Dry it out by covering it with natron (a type of salt) for forty days.
4　Stuff the body with linen or sawdust to give it a life-like shape and sew it up again.
5　Cover the body with scented ointments and coat it with resin.
6　Wrap the body carefully with up to 20 layers of linen sheeting and long bandages. Spells must be said and charms placed in the bandages.
7　The mummy is placed in a sarcophagus or coffin. This is painted with spells and symbols.

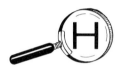

Look at Source G
?　Priest/doctors mummified bodies. How might they have used the knowledge they gained in this process?
?　Does the process of mummification suggest they knew a lot about anything else?

Body-shaped coffins, like that in Source H, could be made from linen, plaster or wood. Often coffins were stacked inside each other. Source H shows a coffin made for a priestess who died in about 1800 BC. It was decorated with pictures to help the priestess on her way to the After-Life. One of these charms was the powerful Eye of Horus. The eye watched for evil spirits and for the route to the After-Life.

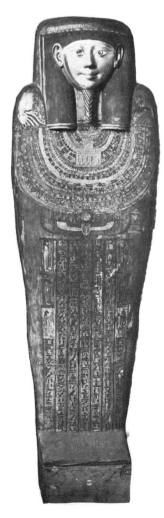

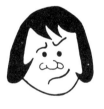

Is that all the medical treatment they used?

No. They were already learning about how the body worked because they had to cut it up to mummify it. The Ebers papyrus and ancient prescriptions tell us that their real medical knowledge was good. The Egyptians invented paper. It was made from reeds that grew in the River Nile. They were papyrus reeds so the paper was called papyrus. It was much thicker and rougher than the writing paper we are used to. What do you think they did to the reeds to make them into papyrus? What sorts of things do you think they wrote on the papyrus? How might these help their passing on medical knowledge?

Egyptian doctors were also priests. We can read about them in the papyri. We can see how they looked after people who were ill. They treated them in Houses of Life. Why do you think doctors were also priests?

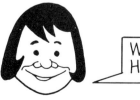

What were Houses of Life?

Houses of life were large temples like the one at Thebes in Egypt, part of which is shown in Source I.

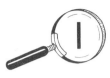

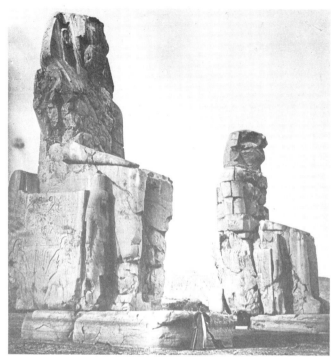

Look at Source I
Behind these statues was a large stone building.
? Why do you think temples like these were so good for sick people?

Proper medical treatment

In the House of Life the priest/doctor gave sick people drugged drinks. The patients then went to sleep. They dreamed, and sometimes they had hallucinations. What are hallucinations?

The priests were paid to say what the dreams meant. They then treated the person who was ill with whatever medicine they needed. Can you think of a Bible story that tells us about someone interpreting the dreams of Pharaoh Ramases II?

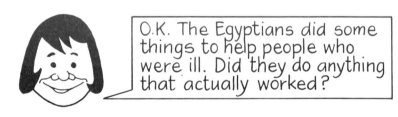

O.K. The Egyptians did some things to help people who were ill. Did they do anything that actually worked?

Yes. They were very careful about keeping clean. They bathed and showered and they washed their hair. They even cleaned their teeth with paste made from sand! All these things are normal to us but remember Egyptians lived thousands of years ago.

They thought pigs were dirty. They would not touch them. Swineherds lived separately from everyone else.

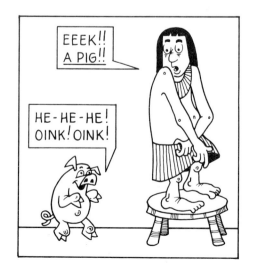

Even though they tried to be clean, evidence from mummies tells us something different. The Egyptians were often badly fed and they had a lot of different kinds of worms and parasites in their bodies. They did not live long. Many of them suffered from all kinds of diseases. Do you think the Egyptians had a dual approach to medicine? Imagine you are a pharaoh living in Ancient Egypt. How would you ensure your body's health in this world and the next?

Other ancient civilisations

There were other ancient civilisations. These were people who lived at the same time as the Egyptians. They lived in other parts of the world.

South America

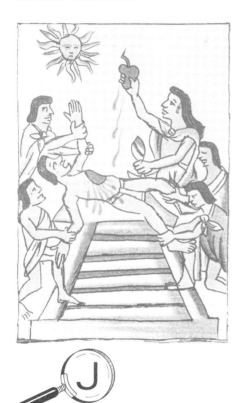

Thousands of years ago there were a lot of communities living in South America. A lot of them thought that there were gods and goddesses looking after them. Does this idea of gods and goddesses remind you of any other people you have looked at? What sort of things do you think they asked the deities for?

Look at Source J
? Describe what you can see in the picture.
? Why do you think someone is being killed?
? Why is the killing done at the top of the steps?
? Who is doing the killing and how?

Source J shows a religious ceremony. The people are worshipping the Sun God. Warriors are being sacrificed. A lot of people in South America prayed to the Sun God. They were called the Incas, the Aztecs and the Mayas. Why do you think the Sun God was so important to them?

They thought the sun lived on blood and heat. Can you think of any reasons why they believed that?

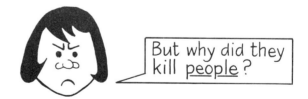

But why did they kill _people_?

The Incas, the Aztecs and the Mayas realised that people died if they lost their blood. They knew that blood was warm and believed that blood carried life around the body. That is why they made human sacrifices to the Sun God. If the Sun God didn't have blood he would die. Do you think they learned anything by sacrificing humans? Make a list of all the things they might have learned.

There were priests who were responsible for killing the sacrificial victim. They were also doctors. These priest/doctors gave their victims pain-killing drinks. They made them from herbs and plants. These drinks were also sedatives.

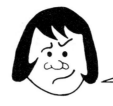

What are sedatives?

Sedatives make a person feel relaxed. Sometimes people who have been given a sedative get very sleepy.

Sedatives can make you feel very giggly and silly. Sometimes your arms and legs don't work properly.

Can you think of any other ways sedatives might have been useful?

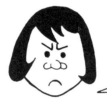

That is all very well but I don't think it helped them much in treating people who are ill.

This is where you are wrong. They found out a lot about anatomy. Use a dictionary to find out what anatomy is. The South American tribes were also clever at making medicines from herbs and plants. They used these to cure people who were ill.

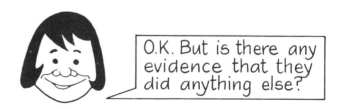

O.K. But is there any evidence that they did anything else?

There is a lot of evidence.
1 There are statues and carvings. These show doctors looking after patients.
2 There are pictures painted on the walls of ancient buildings. Some of these show pictures of hearts and the inside of bodies. They are very accurate. Why might they know a lot about how the heart works as a pump for blood?
3 These are a few documents. These are made from the bark of trees after it has been beaten. In these we can read that the Aztecs did a lot of surgical operations. Can you remember what surgical operations are? The Aztecs were very clever at this. They even used human hair to suture the wound.

Suturing wounds
? What made them decide to use human hair?
? Why was it such a clever idea?

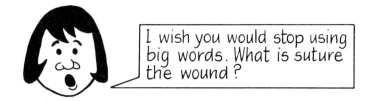

Stitch together the edges of a cut.

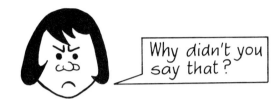

4 The best evidence we have is from Spanish explorers who went to South America from 1540 onwards. They saw the Incas living as they always had done for thousands of years.

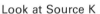

Look at Source K
? How do you think the annual public health festival affected their health?
? Do you think their ideas of dealing with health and preventing illness were clever? Why?
? Is there anything similar that we do today?

Source K

Spanish explorers wrote diaries and log books. They also wrote letters home. Some of these tell that the Incas had a public health festival. This happened every year. The towns were cleared of rubbish and sewage. Houses were thoroughly cleaned. New supplies of fresh water were brought to the town.

South America was not the only place where people knew a lot about medicine. There were other civilisations in other parts of the world who tried to cure illness in a sensible way.

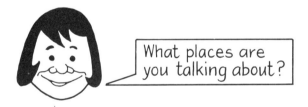

China

China, India and Babylon. We have a lot of evidence about these places. There are documents, paintings, drawings and the ruins of buildings. Try to find out as much background information as you can about all these places.

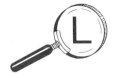

Chinese medicine was very advanced. Acupuncture was just one of their treatments for illness. It is still used today. It involves sticking needles into certain parts of the body to stop pain and cure illness. Very old Chinese jars have been discovered that still contain the remains of herbs and plants. These had been used as medicines or ointments. Do acupuncture and herbal medicine have anything in common?

Look at Source L
? What does it show?
? Why do you think this method of treatment would work?
? Why is acupuncture still used today and what for?

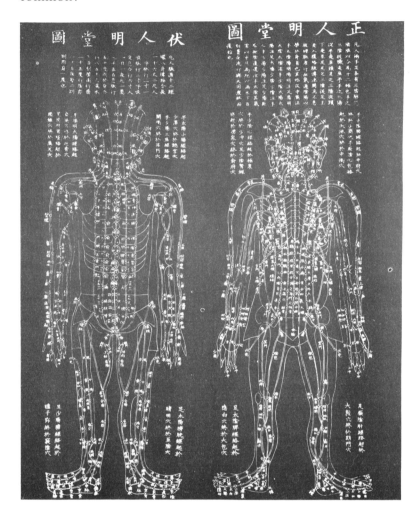

India

India had a very good system of hospitals. It was, perhaps, the first ancient civilisation to have hospitals that we would recognise. They were like modern hospitals in some ways. There are documents about the hospital at Susrata. These show how the hospital was organised. Doctors were properly trained. The doctors could be fined for poor work. Why do you think they were fined as a punishment for bad work? What sort of things might have been judged to be bad work?

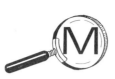

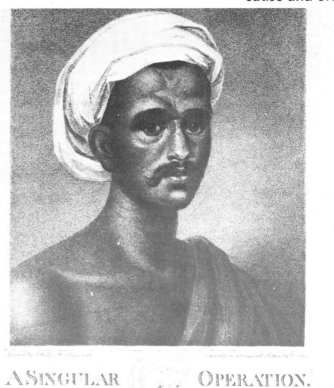

A SINGULAR OPERATION.

Look at Source M
? What does it tell us about
  medicine in India?
? Why were operations like these
  necessary?

Herbs and spices also played a very important part in healing the sick in India. List any reasons why.

Babylon

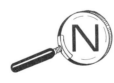

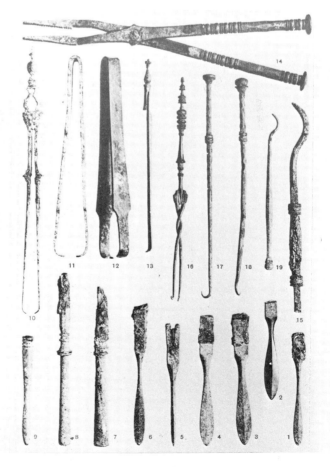

Look at Source N
? What are these?
? What do they tell us about
  medical knowledge in
  Babylon?

Ancient Greece

Key ideas

The ideas of individuals are important.

Individual people's ideas can influence others.

Realistic treatments continue.

Preventative medicine continues.

Search for scientific knowledge.

The people of Ancient Greece

The people who lived in Ancient Greece were called the Greeks. Look at a map of the world. Find out where Greece is. It is a warm country. It has quite a lot of rain. What kinds of food do you think the Greeks ate? Would they have had to hunt for food like Stone Age people? Would this affect the way they lived? How?

The Greeks settled down in places that they liked. Life was much easier. They had far more time. How do you think they used this time?

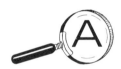

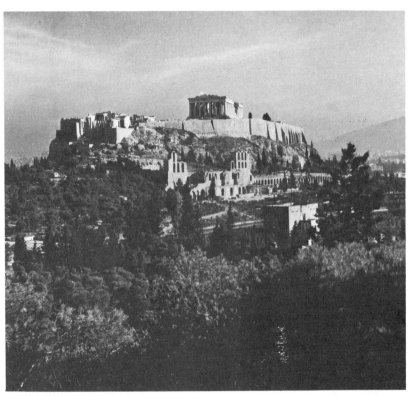

They built beautiful cities like that in Source A. They loved art and nature. They wanted to find out as much about everything as they could. They had time for sport. The first Olympic Games were held in Greece in 776 BC. Source B shows a Greek discus thrower. The original statue was made in 450 BC.

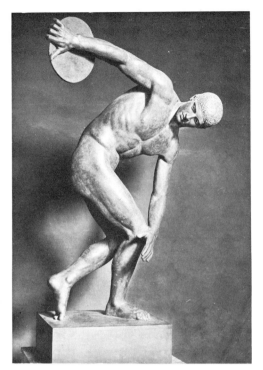

Look at Source B
? What does it tell us about the Greeks' knowledge of the human body?
? What does it show about the Greeks' attitude to fitness?
? How did sculptors make such life-like statues? What must they have known about?

The Greeks wanted to find out about everything. They wanted to know what the world was made of. They wanted to discover why certain things happened, like earthquakes and the seasons. They wanted to know all about illness.

The Greeks believed in gods and goddesses. What might these deities have looked after? The Greeks had a lot of stories and myths to explain things that happened. Their explanation for the seasons of the year was found in the story of Demeter and her daughter Persephone. Demeter's daughter was taken away by the god Zeus. She was allowed home for a certain time every year. When this happened everything was warm. It was sunny and light. Plants grew. Persephone brought spring and summer with her. When she went back to Zeus everything was cold and miserable. This was autumn and winter.

Why did the Greeks make statues of their gods?

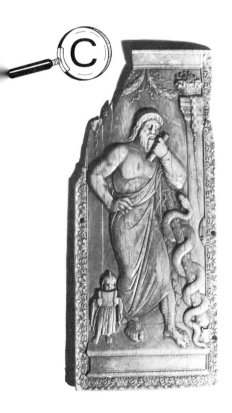

Source C shows a Greek God called Asclepios. His story is found in Greek myths. He was clever at healing people who were ill. We might have called him a doctor. Another Greek God, Pluto, was jealous of Asclepios. He persuaded Zeus to kill Asclepios with a thunderbolt. When he did, Asclepios became a god.

Look at Source C
? How is Asclepios dressed? What is he holding? What is wrapped round it?
? What words would you use to describe Asclepios?
? Why do you think he is shown in this way?
? Why did the Greeks believe that an ordinary doctor like Asclepios could become a God?

What good was Asclepios once he had become a god? Could he still cure people?

Yes. The Greeks built temples to worship Asclepios. A ruin of a temple for Asclepios can still be seen at Epidaurus in Greece. Source D shows Epidaurus. People who were ill would go to pray in the temple of Asclepios. Find the temple in Source D.

Look at Source D
? What do you think the temple looked like inside and out?
? What do you think the temple was built of?
? What buildings show that the Greeks believed in physical fitness?
? What sort of sports might have taken place in the stadium?
? Do any of the buildings show the Greeks believed in the power of the Gods?

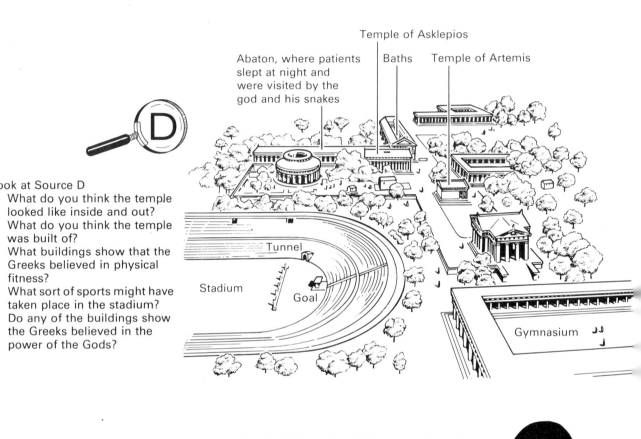

Abaton, where patients slept at night and were visited by the god and his snakes

Temple of Asklepios

Baths

Temple of Artemis

Tunnel

Stadium

Goal

Gymnasium

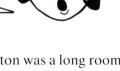

Is that all the people did? Prayed to Asclepios to make them better?

No. They went to the abaton to sleep. The abaton was a long room full of beds. Find it in Source D. We have a modern version of the abaton today. You would find it in hospitals. What is it called?

The importance of Asclepios

While the sick people were sleeping in the abaton, Asclepios was supposed to visit each person. He had with him his two daughters. Source E shows Asclepios and his daughters looking after a patient. The daughter's names were Hygeia and Panacea.

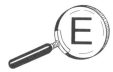

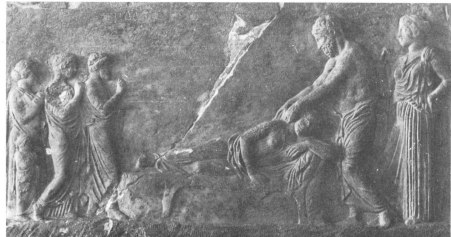

Look at Source E
? What name do we give to the job Hygeia and Panacea are doing?
? What words come from the names of the two daughters? Find out what they mean.

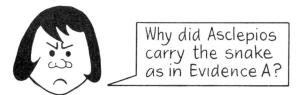

Why did Asclepios carry the snake as in Evidence A?

To cure his patients, Asclepios rubbed their bodies and eyelids with special oil. The snake licked the oil off. When the patients woke up they were supposed to be cured.

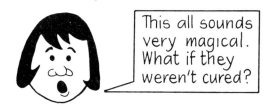

This all sounds very magical. What if they weren't cured?

They stayed at the temple. The temples became more like health clubs or convalescent homes. There was a holiday atmosphere. There were exciting things to do. It might have been the first attempt to stop people becoming ill. It might have cured patients by natural methods like rest and relaxation.

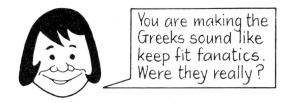

You are making the Greeks sound like keep fit fanatics. Were they really?

Yes. They believed in the healing powers of their gods. They also believed that they should help themselves by eating good food, taking exercise and keeping clean. This was a new approach to medicine.

Teachers and philosophers

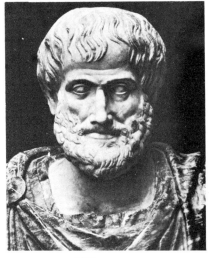

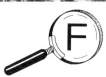

To the Ancient Greeks the need to find out about everything was very important. The people who tried to discover things about science, music, art and medicine were called philosophers. One famous philosopher was Aristotle. You can see a statue of him in Source F.

Aristotle went to Mytilene in Lesbos in 347 BC to study medicine. He cut up the bodies of animals to find out how they worked. This is called dissection. He made some mistakes. He thought people were exactly the same inside as the animals he dissected. This was not always true.

He learned a lot about treating people who were ill. He was an expert at resetting broken bones. He had his own favourite cures for stomach problems. These cures were quite successful.

He believed in a theory that many Greek philosophers and doctors had written about for many years. To them this theory explained the cause of illness. To us it might appear silly. Unfortunately Aristotle and many others believed it was correct. This belief continued for hundreds of years.

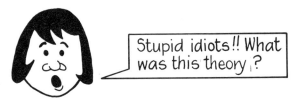

The theory was written about as early as 500 BC by Alcmaeon of Cronton. He was a philosopher and doctor. The theory was as follows.

The idea was that if anything went wrong with your body it was because everything that made up your body was out of balance. They believed that the humours were not balanced correctly. Look at table G. It will help to explain the Four Humours theory.

Table G. The Four Humours

Four Elements	Air	Fire	Earth	Water
Four Seasons	Spring	Summer	Autumn	Winter
Which were	Moist	Hot	Dry	Cold
Similarly There were Four Humours	Sanguine (Hopeful Confident)	Choleric (Angry)	Melancholic (Miserable)	Phlegmatic (Sluggish, Apathetic)
Depending on these liquids in the body	Blood	Yellow bile	Black bile	Phlegm
Leading to these human characteristics	Passionate Active Emotional	Angry, Ill-Tempered	Sad Gloomy Dreamy	Unexciting Dull Even-tempered

If you had too much of one thing you would become ill. For instance, too much yellow bile would make you ill and 'angry'. To put this right a doctor would have given you something to make you vomit. This would have got rid of some of the yellow bile and 'anger'. The balance would be corrected.

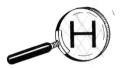

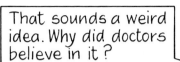

That sounds a weird idea. Why did doctors believe in it?

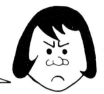

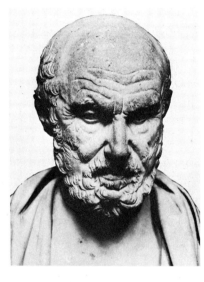

They believed it because they had no other way to explain illness. They did not know anything about germs causing illness. They just believed in something that seemed to make sense. The Four Humours theory showed a reason for illness. It showed why there were certain symptoms like being sick, coughing and sneezing.

Greek ideas lived on for a great many centuries. There was one Greek who tried a more sensible approach to healing. This was Hippocrates. He is called **the father of modern medicine.** His portrait is shown in Source H.

Hippocrates was born on the Greek island of Cos in 460 BC. He travelled a lot. He gained a lot of medical experience. He believed in the Four Humours theory and wrote about it and its use with patients. He also tried a new and original way of treating illness.

1   He observed symptoms.
2   He took notes and records.
3   He used the notes and observations to diagnose his patient's illness.

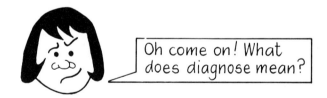

Oh come on! What does diagnose mean?

It means to say exactly what was wrong with someone.

The treatments that Hippocrates used for his patients were fresh air, good food and exercise. These treatments allowed nature to work. Hippocrates was very successful in treating patients with these methods. These cures show a move away from magic.

Hippocrates also wrote a code of behaviour for doctors. It is still used today. It is called the Hippocratic Oath and all new doctors have to take this oath. Source I shows one part of the oath.

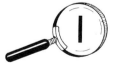

Look at Source I
?   Put this small section of the Hippocratic Oath into your own words. What does it mean?
?   Why is Hippocrates called 'the Father of modern medicine?' Do you agree with the title? Why?

Source I
'In whatever homes I enter . . . I will help the sick and abstain from all intentional wrong doing and harm . . . and whatsoever I shall see or hear . . . I will never divulge.'

The Romans

Key ideas

Roman empire building and its influence.

Changes the Romans introduced.

How far these changes affected medical development.

Evaluating the changes and the effects they had.

The Roman Empire is built

About 2000 years ago Rome was the main city in a very big empire. What is an empire? Rome is in Italy. It is on a river that leads to the Mediterranean Sea, so the people who lived there could travel abroad fairly easily. How do you think Rome's position helped in making it the centre of an empire? It was also part of the mainland of Europe. What methods of transport might you have used if you had lived in Rome 2000 years ago?

The leaders of Rome were often good at governing and organising. They wanted beautiful buildings like the one in Source A.

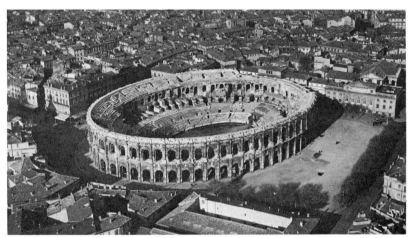

Look at Source A
? What skills would the Romans have needed to construct buildings like these?
? What does this source of evidence tell us about the Romans?

The Romans tried to copy the Greeks. They tried to build like the Greeks. They tried to govern in the same way as the Greeks had. The Romans also believed in learning as much as possible about everything.

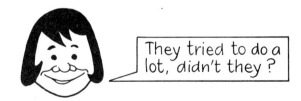

They tried to do a lot, didn't they?

Yes, but they soon found out that it cost them a lot of money. They also needed a lot of people to work for them. How do you think they got money to build their empire? Where would they find enough people to work for them? How might they have persuaded people to work for them?

? What changes might the Roman army have made in the Roman Empire? Why?

To get people and money the Romans had a very powerful army. There were several ranks in the **Roman Army**. There were centurions on horseback. The standard bearer had the important job of carrying the legion's flag or standard. The ordinary foot soldiers were called legionaries. The lowest ranks were the auxiliaries.

The Roman soldiers were well trained and were very fit. They could march up to 40 miles every day. They built roads to make their journeys easier. You can see a Roman road in Source B.

Look at Source B
? What do the Roman roads look like? What are they made of?
? Do you think they were good roads? Why?
? What changes would the roads have made to the Roman Empire?
? Would anyone else have benefited from the roads besides the army?

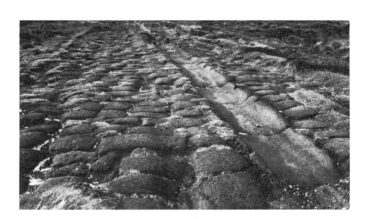

The Romans also built bridges, forts, walls and many other things. These helped them to win many battles and get land from other people. The Romans brought many other countries under the rule of the Roman Empire.

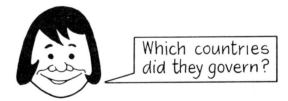

Which countries did they govern?

Italy, Germany, France, Spain, North Africa, parts of Egypt, Persia, Syria and England.

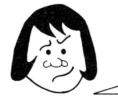

That's a lot of countries. I suppose they invaded so many to get wealth and workers. Were the names the same 2000 years ago?

Not always. France was called Gaul by the Romans. England was called the Dark Land of Mists.

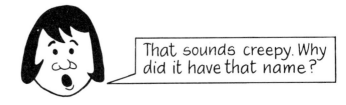

That sounds creepy. Why did it have that name?

The Romans in Britain

England could just be seen across the foggy sea we now call the English Channel. It didn't have much contact with the rest of Europe. The people who lived there were supposed to be wild and dangerous.

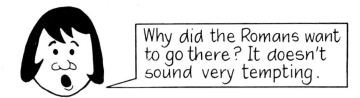

Why did the Romans want to go there? It doesn't sound very tempting.

Julius was the Roman Emperor in 54 BC. He was called Julius Caesar. All Roman Emperors added Caesar to their names. He needed men to build the Empire and join his army. He needed slaves to serve the Roman people. Julius Caesar also needed gold. He thought he might find all of these things in England so he came to conquer it with his army. Imagine you were a soldier with Julius Caesar's army. How would you have felt about going to this strange, mysterious island across the sea?

When the Romans came to Britain they didn't have an easy time. The groups or tribes of people who lived in England hated them. The famous Queen Boudicca of the Iceni tribe in East Anglia, fought the Romans but when she lost she killed herself and her daughters. This was because she did not want to be captured by the Romans. Her statue can be seen in London. Did the Roman invasion affect the lives of people in Britain? If so, how?

The people in Britain fought back, so the Romans had to build forts and walls to protect the land they won. They built two enormous walls across the country to keep out the dangerous tribes in the north. These tribes were called the Picts and the Scots. One wall, the Antonine Wall, was soon destroyed. The other wall was bigger and stronger. It stretched from one side of England to the other. It was called Hadrian's Wall and it can still be seen today.

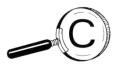

Look at Source C
? What is Hadrian's Wall made from?
? How have the Romans used the natural features of the land?
? Why were huge ditches dug on either side of the wall?
? Do you think it worked in keeping out enemies?
? In what way did the wall affect the people already living there?

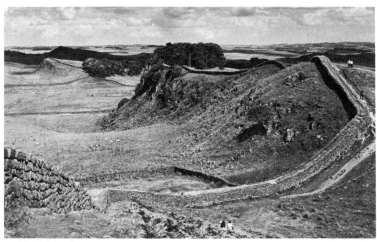

A soldier's life

Along Hadrian's Wall archaeologists have discovered several forts built as part of the wall to house the Roman guards. The two most famous are Housesteads and Vindolanda. The remains of these forts tell us a lot about the Roman's medicine and ideas about health and hygiene.

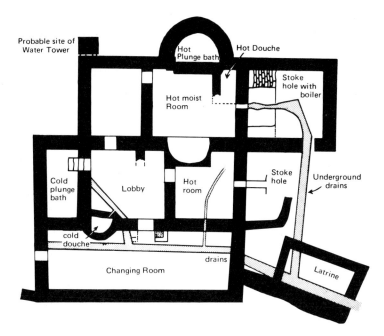

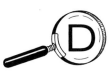

Look at Source D
? What do these buildings tell us about Roman soldiers serving in Britain?
? What is the latrine? Why is it so important?
? Why do you think the latrine was built so near to the bath house?

Source D shows the bath-house at Housesteads. There was also a large, well-equipped hospital. It was a square building with several rooms round an open courtyard. Doctors and medical orderlies helped sick soldiers. What sort of illness or injury might the doctors have had to deal with? Some of the doctors were young Greeks who wanted to gain practical experience. Why do you think there were Greek doctors with the Roman army? The writings of a Roman called Pliny tell us that these army doctors knew a lot about herbal medicine and sensible medical treatments for injury. Do you think that these doctors also treated the Britons who were living in the area?

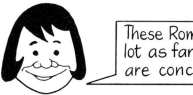

These Romans sound a promising lot as far as health and hygiene are concerned.

Public health

Source E shows the remains of the latrines at Housesteads. Source F shows an artist's idea of what the latrines would have been like when the Romans occupied Housesteads.

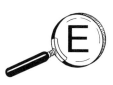

Look at Sources E and F
? Describe the latrines. In what ways are they different from public toilets today?
? How were the Roman latrines flushed?
? Where did the sewage go to?
? Did the Romans have toilet paper? If not, what did they have?
? Where did they wash?

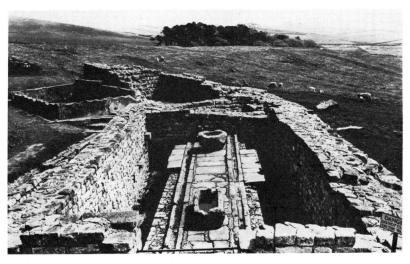

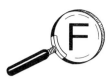

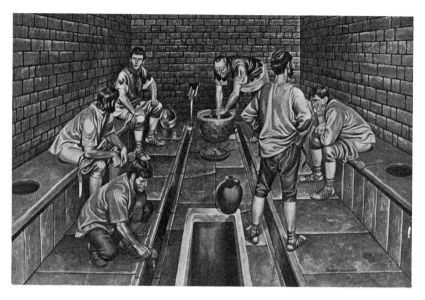

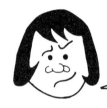

That all sounds very public and uncomfortable. Were these the only toilets in the Roman Empire?

No. There are many remains of Roman latrines all over the area covered by the Roman Empire. There are some very good examples in North Africa. They are very similar to the latrines at Housesteads. By AD 315 the city of Rome itself had 144 public latrines, all flushed with running water.

The Romans built sewers in all their big towns and cities. They were round and built of stone or brick, and were so good they lasted for hundreds of years. The ones in Rome were still used as sewers until World War II in 1939. Do these ideas about sanitation tell you anything about the Romans? What do we have today similar to the Roman ideas?

If you look back to Source D you will see that Housesteads had baths for its soldiers. The Romans enjoyed many sports and leisure activities. The most popular of these was their time spent at the public baths. In England there is an excellent example of Roman baths at the city of Bath in Avon (look at Source G). The Romans called the city Aquae Sulis. Aquae means water in Latin, which was the language spoken by the Romans. The public baths were so well built that parts of them are in working order today.

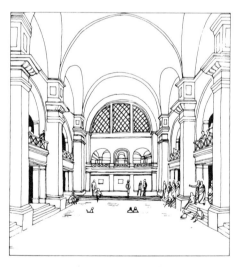

The baths

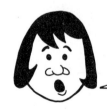

What happened at the baths? Did the Romans just go swimming?

No. It was far more complicated than that.

First they undressed. Then all the hair was plucked off their bodies by slaves with tweezers. Next they were massaged with oil. This was then scraped off with a curved instrument called a strigil, which took the dirt and sweat off their bodies. They could then go to the gymnasium to exercise, play games, do weight lifting and wrestling. They could relax. There was a music room and a room where they could get food and drink. There was a steam room like a modern sauna and a large swimming pool. There was also an ice-cold plunge. Lastly they went to a warm room where they could relax and get dressed.

? Imagine yourself having a day at the baths in Roman times. Describe what happened to you during the day.

? How did the baths affect the lives of Romans living in Britain? Do you think other people adopted their ideas? Why?

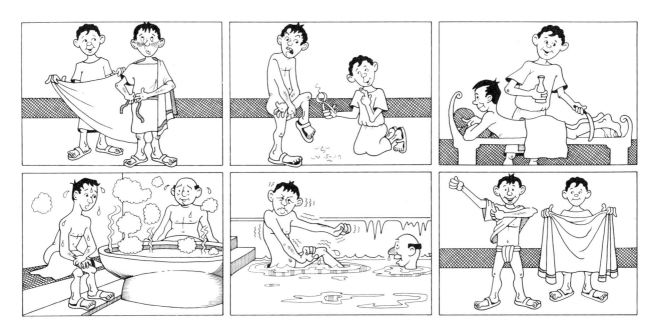

Engineering and building

To get baths just where and how they wanted the Romans had to do two things. They had to pipe water quite long distances. They had to be able to heat water and certain rooms. The Romans built water pipes of bricks, usually lined with lead. They built canals. The Romans constructed aqueducts to carry water over mountains and valleys. They built huge cisterns to supply their towns and villas with water. Source H shows the Roman aqueduct at Nimes. It is still in use today.

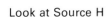

Look at Source H
? Would this fresh water supply change the lives of the Romans at all? List any possible changes.
? Were there any problems with their ideas and constructions?

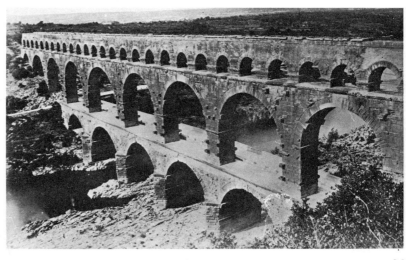

The Romans used central heating systems, which they invented. Buildings had furnaces under the main floor. Air ducts were built and were lined with special tiles. These ducts carried hot air around the buildings. Why would central heating be needed? Who would keep the furnace burning? Which houses in Britain would benefit from the central heating?

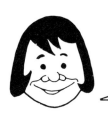

So the Romans had toilets which flushed. They had sewers. They had running water. They were particular about keeping clean. The Romans took exercise and kept fit.

Medical knowledge

Yes. They also took care about where they built their towns and villas. A Roman leader called Marcus Varro suggested a country life for everyone. He said that towns should be built on wooded hillsides 'with health-giving winds'. The Romans realised that swamps and mosquitoes usually caused illness. They had recognised the link between mosquitoes and malaria. They drained swamps and tried to avoid living near them. They also built temples to Febris, the goddess of the swamps to protect themselves. Does this show that the Romans had a dual approach to medicine?

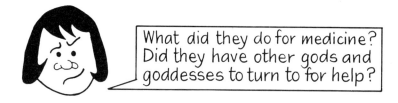

What did they do for medicine? Did they have other gods and goddesses to turn to for help?

Yes. They prayed to deities for protection against illness. The main temple was at Delphi, which was an island in the river Tiber at Rome. A sacred snake was supposed to have swum ashore there. A temple was built for the sick and was looked after by an oracle.

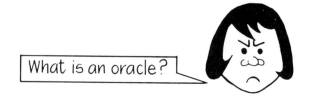

What is an oracle?

A kind of priest who gave advice about treating illness. The temple eventually became more like a modern hospital with wards, doctors and nurses. The Romans not only believed in gods, they had practical ideas about treating illness. There were a lot of military hospitals at the forts. Source I shows a cross section of the military hospital at Inchtuthil in Scotland. The ruins of this building can still be seen.

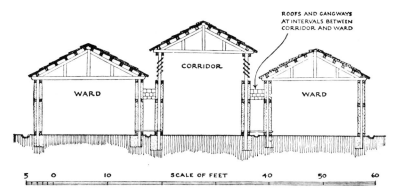

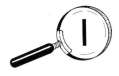

Look at Source I
? In what ways is this hospital like modern hospitals?
? Why did forts need hospitals?

Doctors and knowledge

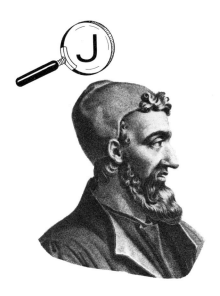

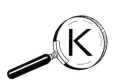

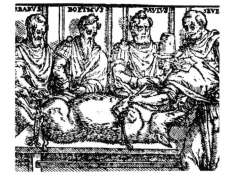

Look at Source K
? Why did Galen make mistakes about anatomy?
? Did Galen help the development of medicine or did he hold it back?

The army doctors were always dealing with soldiers wounded in battle. They often found out about the inside of the body this way. Some surgeons were very skillful. They removed tumours, set broken bones and even tried skin grafting. Today we call this plastic surgery. Discuss with your teacher what this involves. When would a doctor need to try skin grafting?

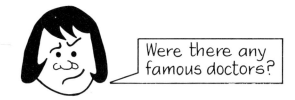

Were there any famous doctors?

Yes. Dioscorides was a very important doctor. He believed in using herbs to make medicines. He used these to treat illness. He travelled all over the world finding out about herbs and plants and how to use them. He wrote a book called 'Herbarium'. It was used for hundreds of years.

Even more famous was a doctor called Galen. He is shown in Source J and in Source K.

He travelled through many countries. He learned a lot about anatomy by dissecting animals. He is shown dissecting a pig in Source K. He made a lot of mistakes because he thought people were made just like animals. Unfortunately his ideas lasted until 1628.

Galen believed that 'spirit' was breathed in and mixed with blood in the heart. This was carried to the brain. It then went round the body causing movement and sensation. He believed that God caused this. His beliefs were used by the Christian church for hundreds of years. Galen followed the ideas of the Greeks about illness being caused by the humours. Can you remember the Four Humours theory? Look back to Unit 3 and revise the theory. Galen did some work on the nervous system. He was stubborn and he refused to listen to anyone else's ideas. He tried to use his knowledge in his treatment of illness but his knowledge unfortunately was often wrong.

The Romans brought changes all over their Empire. Occasionally these affected everyone. Often their ideas disappeared when the Romans left. How popular did their ideas become in the countries of the Empire? Did Britain change because of the Romans?

The Dark Ages

Key ideas

Using evidence to find out about medicine in the Dark Ages.

Judging whether the evidence is reliable or not.

Evaluating the evidence.

The importance of monks and the Church in medical development.

The part played by barber-surgeons.

Evidence

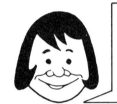

So far we have seen people who lived thousands of years ago. They relied on gods and magic to help them. They also had some real medical treatments. There was some progress. Right?

Right! There were some good ideas. Some treatments worked. List three pieces of evidence that show medical treatments that worked. Are the sources of this evidence likely to be accurate? Can we believe what they tell us? Why? Was medicine improving?

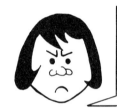

So there was progress! But you've called this Chapter The Dark Ages. That suggests something bad and mysterious. Was it that bad?

This unit is called the Dark Ages for two reasons.

1   There is not much evidence from the years AD 400 to AD 1100. Can you think of any reasons why? If there is not much evidence then it is hard to know exactly what happened. We have to be detectives. We make guesses from the evidence there is. The evidence does not shed much light on these centuries. They are 'dark'.

2   This period is called the Dark Ages because a lot of the people who lived then were not well educated. They couldn't read or write. Most people would never leave the villages and areas where they were born. Ideas spread very slowly. The people relied on the Christian church for nearly everything. There was not much progress.

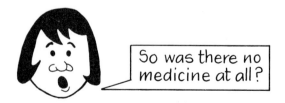

So was there no medicine at all?

Oh yes! There is some evidence to show that good medical ideas were used.

Medicine

Bishop Nestorius of Constantinople was exiled from the Church in Europe. He set up a school of medicine in Persia in AD 431. He was helped by his monks who wrote about it. Is evidence about Nestorius likely to be accurate? Can you think of any reasons why it might be biased?

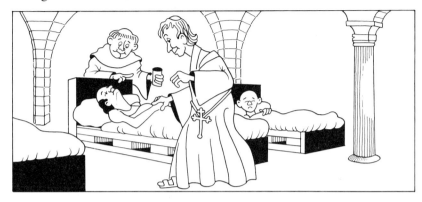

Some monks wrote books by hand in Latin. It took a long time. Some of the books included sections on medicine. The books can be seen in museums today. One such book was 'De Medicina' by the monk Celsus. Do you think these books are a good source of evidence about the past? Why? What problems might historians have in interpreting or translating these books?

Leech books were popular in England from AD 800 onwards. They were written in English but it would be very difficult for us to read. It was very different from our written language. The leech books mention witchcraft, herbalism and leeches. They included many folk-lore remedies. Can you think of any folk-lore remedies we still use today?

Doctors

Leeches were used to suck people's blood. Doctors believed a patient was ill because he had too much blood.

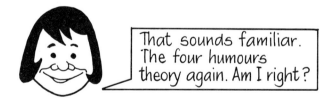

That sounds familiar. The four humours theory again. Am I right?

Yes. The doctor would prescribe leeches. He carried them with him in a leech jar. They were put on the patient's skin. There they would bite and suck the blood.

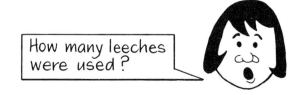

How many leeches were used?

? Imagine you are going to visit a doctor in the middle ages. He is famous for his use of leeches. How would you feel about it?

Sometimes one, sometimes fifteen. It depended on what the doctor said. The doctor put cups over them to make them suck better.

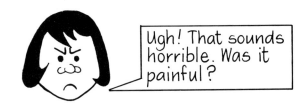

Yes, very. But it was a treatment that was used for hundreds of years.

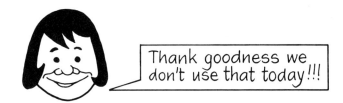

You'd be surprised! In very delicate brain surgery, instruments are sometimes too big. Special small leeches are bred to place in the wound to clear the blood.

There were some trained doctors to help the sick. Source A shows a doctor at work in the Dark Ages.

Look at Source A
? How many people are in the picture?
? Which is the doctor? How do you know?
? Has the doctor got an assistant?
? What is happening to the patient?
? What differences are there between a visit to a doctor in the Dark Ages and a visit to a doctor today?

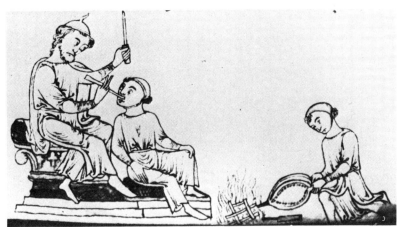

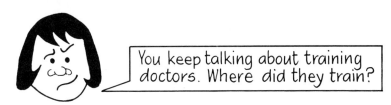

They usually trained at universities and medical schools. Is this the same today? Two famous medical schools were Montpellier and Salerno in France. Monks and civilian men went to these schools.

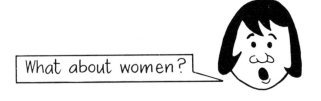

Women were not allowed in schools or universities. Some women trained themselves by reading and studying. Women often knew a lot about herbs. They were the experts when it came to midwifery. But they were **not** encouraged to become doctors. What reasons can you think of for women not being given the same opportunities as men? When a man wanted to become a doctor he went to University for six years to learn about medicine. He only worked with patients for two summers of this time. What does this tell us about his training? Is it the same today? Monks trained to be doctors in the same way. There was a difference though. They lived in monasteries. Sick people went to monasteries for treatment. The monks who were studying to be doctors had contact with sick people a lot of the time. They had real experience. If you were ill would you have gone to a newly qualified doctor?

Monks and medicines

Poor people and travellers could get treatment at the monasteries. Many monastery hospitals had all or some of the following comforts: large size, plenty of monks to treat the sick, heating, pharmacies, windows that could be opened, regular cleaning, fur bed covers, two meals daily. From this list do you think patients were well treated in monasteries? In many places monastery infirmaries were the only hospitals available. List the differences and similarities with hospitals today.

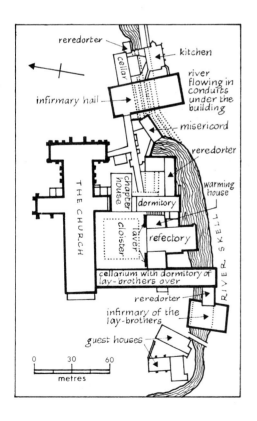

Look at Source B, which shows Fountains Abbey, Yorkshire.
? Where was the infirmary sited? Why?
? How do we know?
? How big is the infirmary compared with the rest of the abbey?
? The hospital was called the infirmary. What do think the monk in charge of the infirmary was called?

In 1130 the Church Council at Clermont banned all churchmen from being doctors or practicing medicine.

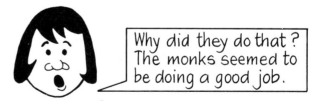

Why did they do that? The monks seemed to be doing a good job.

That's true. But remember, the Church believed that God was in charge of everything. If anyone tried to interfere with illness, they were interfering in God's will. God made people ill. Monks were not allowed to interfere with this.

How long did the ban last?

Not long, thank goodness. Monks were soon practicing medicine again. They came up with some good ideas. A German monk called Nöhter realised the importance of examining patients' urine. This helped him to find out what was the matter with them. This study was called urology. It became very fashionable and it is still important today.

A monk called Rahere travelled all the way to England from Rome. He had been a court jester before he became a monk. He learned a lot about medicine. He founded the famous St Bartholomew's Hospital in London. It is shown in Source C. It is still an important teaching hospital today. Rahere's tomb is in the hospital.

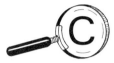

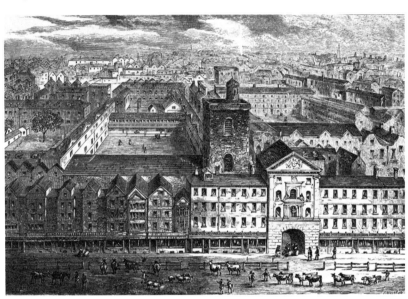

Look at Source C
? Why might a monk be able to found a hospital?
? Would Rahere's earlier career as a court jester help him in the founding of St Bartholomew's hospital?

Barber-surgeons

A barber-surgeon did two jobs. He cut hair and shaved customers. He worked as a doctor. He stopped wounds from bleeding, pulled out teeth and mended broken bones. (Look at Source D.) He taught his apprentices the same things. We can still see Guild Records of Apprentices today. The apprentices were often ill-treated and badly paid. How reliable are these records likely to be?

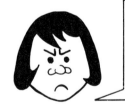

Some of the things that a barber-surgeon did seem pretty horrible... ..and bad for the patient! Still, I suppose they were realistic attempts at treating the sick.

Yes. There was very good work being done in other parts of the world as well.

Arabia was famous for its doctors. Paper had been invented in Egypt. Arabic scholars used it to write translations of medical books. They also wrote many new books. The religion the Arabs followed was Islam. The Arabs attempted to spread the Islamic faith throughout the world. Like the Romans they had an enormous empire. Where Islam spread so did new ideas in medicine.

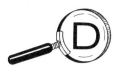

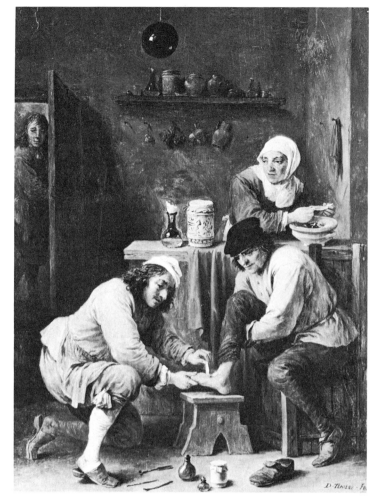

Look at Source D
? Is evidence about barber-surgeons likely to be accurate?
? List the medical treatments the barber-surgeon might have carried out.
? What instruments did he use?
? Why did he often spread disease instead of curing it? How do we know?

Arab doctors – progress

We have evidence about the Arab doctors from books and records they wrote themselves. There are also Arabic pictures and diagrams showing their work. Is this evidence likely to be accurate? Source E shows some famous Arabic doctors.

Source E. Some famous Arabic doctors

Name	What he did
Rhases	He wrote books about hygiene, symptoms, medical treatment, diet. He separated the symptoms of measles and smallpox. He used Plaster of Paris for setting bones. He wrote an encyclopaedia of medicine. He went blind from too much studying.
Avicenna	He wrote books about anatomy and chemistry. He was a hospital supervisor at Damascus and Cairo.
Albucassis	He died aged 101! He wrote the first illustrated book on surgery. He made some mistakes in anatomy because Islam banned dissection of dead bodies.

Look at Source E
? Do you think the chart gives a good overall picture of what they know?
? What problems might historians have had using Arabic medical books as source material?

Monks, doctors and Arab physicians all helped medicine to advance in the Dark Ages. Their work was mostly guess work. When they got something correct it was often by chance. Still, real medicine was improving.

The Middle Ages — epidemics and disease

Key ideas

Fast spread of disease despite poor communications.

Lack of knowledge and ability to fight disease.

Bowing to the will of God.

Effects of disease.

Seeing epidemics from the viewpoint of people at that time.

Diseases

We said that not many people travelled far in the Dark Ages. But one thing travelled a long way. It also travelled very fast. Disease.

A lot of different illnesses were common. Some were not very dangerous. Others were killers. Disease spread quickly from person to person. A disease that does this is called contagious. If the illness affects thousands of people, perhaps even in different countries, it is called an epidemic.

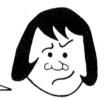

Were there any epidemics which didn't kill many people – just made them ill for a time?

Yes. Influenza and measles were like this. Even then some people died. Why do you think simple diseases like these killed people?

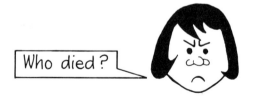

Who died?

Old people and babies died from simple diseases. What reasons can you think of that old people and babies died of what we think of as minor illnesses today?

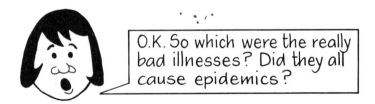

O.K. So which were the really bad illnesses? Did they all cause epidemics?

There were some really dangerous diseases. They killed lots of people.

1 St Anthony's Fire

The real name for this was erysipelas. It was caused by eating bread made with rye that had fungus growing on it. Rye that was stored for later use often became mouldy. Every peasant ate rye bread so a lot of them suffered from this disease. Why were most of the people who caught this disease poor people?

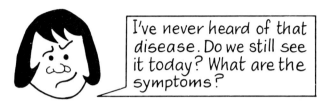

I've never heard of that disease. Do we still see it today? What are the symptoms?

Votive offerings
? Do you think it was a good idea to leave limbs in the church as an offering? Why?
? Could people really avoid catching St Anthony's Fire?

We mostly find it in animals today. Occasionally people suffer from it. In the Middle Ages it caused ulcers on the arms and legs. The skin would sometimes rot away. In very bad cases the limb would sometimes fall off! If the person survived he would take the limb or a model of it to his local church. This was called a votive offering.

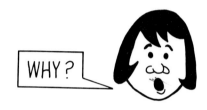

WHY?

It was an offering to God. A 'thank-you' for making the person well again.

2 St Vitus Dance

This was a disease that affected the nerves and muscles. An affected person no longer had control of his body. His limbs made odd jerking movements. This illness still exists today. There is a carving in Echternach in Luxemburg on the tomb of St Willibrod that shows a procession of people with St Vitus Dance. They are praying for help.

? Do you think the carving on the tomb at Echternach in Luxemburg shows that there was still a dual approach to medicine? How?
? Source A shows a man with leprosy. Can you see what it has done to his hands?

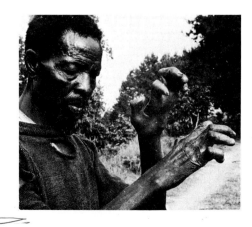

3 Leprosy

This disease still exists in the world today. Doctors are beginning to fight it and win. They know that it is caused by a germ called a bacillus that gets into the blood stream. It attacks the nerves in a person's body. The damage causes loss of all feeling in that part of the body. The usual attack points are the fingers, toes and nose. These get damaged because they are numb, the blood supply is affected and so they rot away and sometimes fall off. The effect of this is horrible to look at. Doctors today fight the disease with drugs. They know the cause of the disease so they are successful in fighting it. In the Middle Ages no one knew how it was caused. People believed it was a punishment from God. Lepers were thought of as evil and unclean. They were banished from their homes. They lived in leper colonies. As they travelled to these colonies they had to ring a bell and shout 'unclean' to warn people to keep away from them.

Look at Source B
? What do you think life must have been like for somebody suffering from leprosy? How did they find food and shelter? How would they have felt about their miserable life?

The Black Death — how it spread

Source B is from the book *Papillon* and tells of leper colonies in the 1930s.

Source B

'Very close to me . . . one of them sat down and it was then I saw my first leper's face. It was horrible and I made an effort not to turn away or show what I felt. His nose was entirely eaten away, a hole right in the middle of his face. Only one ear. His right hand still had two fingers.'

4 The Plague

This disease was the worst killer in the Middle Ages. There were two really bad epidemics in England. One was in 1348 and the other was in 1665. This disease was usually called the Black Death.

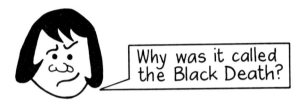

There were two reasons. It was spread by fleas, which lived on black rats. The disease often caused large black lumps or spots on a person's body.

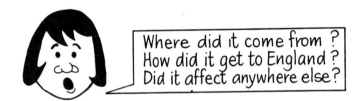

The black rats lived in China. In about AD 1200 explorers from Europe discovered China. They called it Cathay. Name one explorer you may have heard of who got to China. When the ships docked in China the rats were attracted on board by the spices and food in the cargo holds. How do you think the rats got on board? How could the sailors try to prevent the rats getting on the ships?

The ships sailed for Europe with the rats on board. These rats had fleas. The fleas lived on the rats' blood. The blood contained the plague germs.

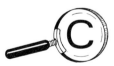

Look at Source C
? This is an enlarged picture of a flea. What do you notice about its back legs? How would these legs help fleas to spread the plague?
? What do you notice about the mouth of the flea? How did it use its mouth?

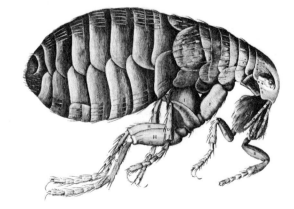

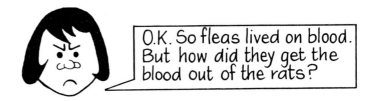

O.K. So fleas lived on blood. But how did they get the blood out of the rats?

You should be able to see a long tube at the mouth of the flea in Source C. This is called a proboscis. The flea bites the rat. It pushes the tube into the wound. It pours its own saliva down the tube to keep the rat's blood flowing. It then sucks the blood. The plague germs are transferred into the flea.

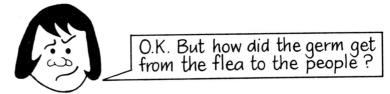

O.K. But how did the germ get from the flea to the people?

In those days people knew nothing about germs. They had no microscopes. They couldn't see germs so they didn't know germs existed. They didn't know that germs love dirt. The people in the Middle Ages were very dirty. They lived in poor houses that were more like huts. They shared these with animals. They had no toilets. They had no water supply except the stream or well. The conditions that people lived in made them an easy target for disease.

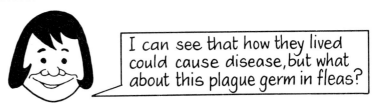

I can see that how they lived could cause disease, but what about this plague germ in fleas?

When ships docked after leaving China the rats often got off the ships to find more food. They would go into the town. They could actually live in the walls of the houses, which were made of wood, straw, mud and animal dung. The fleas were fussy whose blood they lived on, but if the rats died from the plague infection, they would jump off the rats and onto the people.

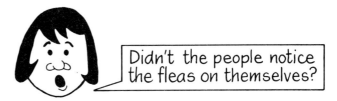

Didn't the people notice the fleas on themselves?

No. Why didn't they notice them? What do you think happened when the fleas bit people?

The ships carrying plague rats left China in about 1345–6. The first place that plague spread to was Italy. Why do you think Italy was the first country affected? The plague hit England in 1348. It was brought ashore by two sailors. Where do you think they had come from? The rats also came ashore. The fleas could now affect more people.

Effects of the Black Death

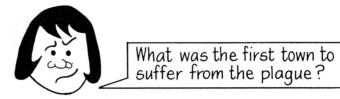

What was the first town to suffer from the plague?

Melcombe Regis in Dorset.

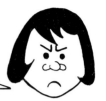

How do you know?

We know from parish records and registers. These tell us about burials and sometimes the reasons for death. Source D shows parish records from Aylesbury in Buckinghamshire. They were written by Robert Lenthall. He was the parish priest.

Source D

'My daughter Sarah Lenthall was buried the eleventh day of August . . . She was aged 14 years, eleven months and seventeen days. Susanna Lenthall my wife departed this life . . . the 26th of August . . . and was buried near her daughter Sarah.
John Gardiner, a child that lived in my house died . . . and was buried August 29th.
Adrian Lenthall, my son . . . near one and twenty years of age . . . was buried at the head of his sister's grave.'

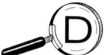

Look at Source D
? Which people died of the plague?
? What effects did the plague have on (a) families, (b) villages, (c) the whole country?
? Why did the parish priest write the records?

It is quite easy to find out where the plague was in England. The Parish records kept in most churches go back hundreds of years. These show the dates of people's burials and sometimes show what they died from. By reading the church records and looking at grave-stones, historians have discovered that the plague arrived in Melcombe Regis in May. By August it had reached London. It was still spreading through the winter and reached the northern parts of England in early 1349. It slowly died out then and only a few cases are recorded in Scotland. In the outbreak in 1665 the progress of the plague is easier to trace. It stayed mainly in London and the South of England but the effects were the same.

By the time the plague had finished in 1349 between half and two-thirds of the population of England was dead. This would be like a nuclear war today. The number of people affected was enormous.

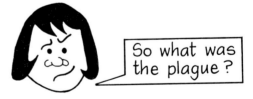

So what was the plague?

The symptoms

The Black Death was really three different kinds of plague. They all come from the same germ but were spread and affected people in different ways.
The three types of plague were:
1 Bubonic, which caused lumps and spots.
2 Septicaemic, which poisoned the blood.
3 Pneumonic, which affected the breathing.

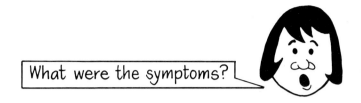

What were the symptoms?

Lumps or spots appeared. These were usually near the joints, especially the groin and the armpits. The victim would be very hot or very cold. This is called a fever. The person might sneeze or cough a lot. They would vomit. Often they would cough up blood. If a person caught the disease they could be dead in less than a day. The usual survival time was about three days. Very few people were ever cured.

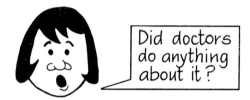

Did doctors do anything about it?

Not really. Source E shows what an Italian writer called Boccacio wrote, in 1348, in his book 'The Decameron'.

Look at Source E
? Where did Boccacio say the disease started?
? In his opinion what two things caused the disease?
? How many people did he say died?
? Did Boccacio think the disease could be beaten?
? What was his opinion of doctors?

Source E
'It started in the East, either through the influence of heavenly bodies or because of God's just anger with our wicked deeds sent it as a punishment to mortal men and in a few years killed an inumerable quantity of people. Ceaselessly passing from place to place, it extended its miserable length over the west. Against this plague all human wisdom and foresight were vain. No doctor's advice, no medicine could overcome or alleviate the disease.'

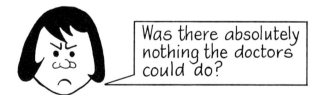

Was there absolutely nothing the doctors could do?

Attempting cures

They tried some cures. Sniffing a posy of flowers was thought to prevent the spread of the disease. Most of you may know the children's nursery rhyme in Source F. It comes from the time of the Black Death.

Look at Source F
? What do you think it all means?
? How were posies of flowers supposed to help matters?

Source F
Ring o' ring o' roses,
A pocket full of posies.
Atishoo, atishoo,
We all fall down.

Other cures were attempted. Hot onions were placed in the patient's ears or armpits. Do you think they did any good? Why? Dried toads were placed on the black lumps on a person's body. When they swelled up with pus from the boils they were replaced. How effective do you think this was?

Some doctors tried to con their rich patients by taking gold and precious stones from them. They said that these treasures could be ground down to a powder. This powder was supposed to be put in the rich victim's drink. Often the powder was just chalk or even bones. What do you think happened to the treasures?

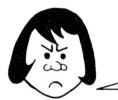

All these so called cures are ridiculous! Did anyone try anything sensible?

Yes. One doctor in France was trying real cures that actually worked. His name was Guy de Chauliac. His main treatment was to cut open the black lumps on patient's bodies. The pus inside was drained out. The wounds were washed with wine. This cleaned and disinfected them. Some of his patients survived.

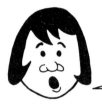

It must have been terrible to live in England during these epidemics.

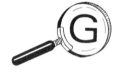

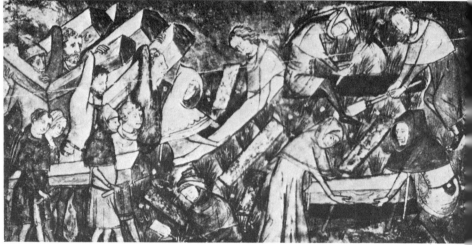

It certainly was terrible to experience the epidemics. At the beginning of the epidemic people were buried properly in coffins. By the later stages bodies were thrown into lime pits outside towns. This was to get rid of them as soon as possible. What other reasons were there for the bodies not being buried properly?

The same thing happened during the 1665 outbreak of the Black Death. The cry heard at night in towns and cities was 'Bring out your dead'. Whole families were sealed up in their own homes with plague victims. Their doors were marked with a cross. They had the words 'Lord have mercy upon us' written on them.

Life during the Plague

Source H shows scenes from 1665. The scenes show the conditions during the plague. Some people blamed God. Some people blamed witchcraft and the devil. Some blamed the stars and heavenly bodies. Nobody thought to blame germs and dirt.

Thousands of people died. Villages were deserted. Animals were left to roam or die. Crops were left to rot. Whole families died whether they were rich or poor. Try to imagine what life must have been like for a person living in a village in England during that time.

1 Write a conversation between a doctor and the town mayor when they find out that the Black Death has reached a village just five miles away.

2 Describe your village and the things that happened there during the plague. You survived. Did your family?

Look at Source H
? How are the bodies being buried?
? How were the bodies taken away?
? How did people know that the plague has reached the town? How did they know which families were affected?
? Families suffering from the disease had 'God have mercy' written on their door. Why do you think this happened?
? Plague families' doors were sealed. How do you think they got food?

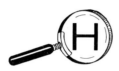

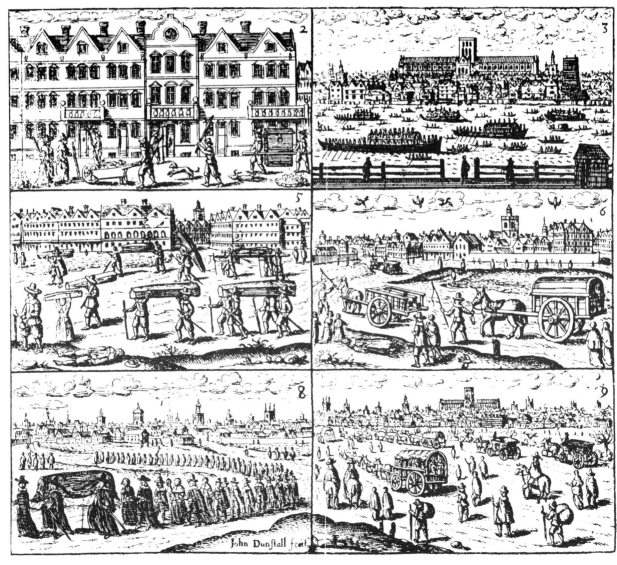

John Dunstall fecit

The Renaissance

Key ideas

New ideas and discoveries were made.

Old ideas persisted.

The effect of the Church on change and new ideas.

What was the Renaissance?

The word 'Renaissance' means reborn. At this time people became more interested in new ideas. They were also interested in old books and ideas. Many of these ideas came from Greek books.

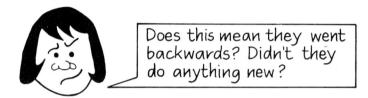

Does this mean they went backwards? Didn't they do anything new?

Yes, they did. The people were interested in science and art. They enjoyed poetry and literature. The people were also beginning to ask if God really existed. Why were people starting to question the existence of God?

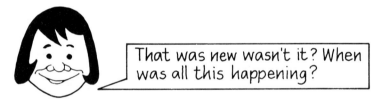

That was new wasn't it? When was all this happening?

The Renaissance was from about AD 1350 to AD 1650. There were a lot of ideas, especially in science and art, but old ideas still continued despite new knowledge.

Science

The telescope was invented. A scientist in Italy called Galileo developed and made telescopes and used them to see stars and planets. Most people believed the world was flat like a plate. If you went far enough you would fall off the edge. Galileo's telescopes provided evidence to support the idea that the world was round. He believed the world floated in space and moved round the sun. He got into trouble with the Church for these new ideas. All his books were burnt. Why do you think the church did not like Galileo's ideas? Why did the Church punish him by burning his books?

Art

Before the Renaissance most artists painted scenes from the Bible. Their main job was to decorate churches and palaces. The people they painted were not very life-like. Can you think of any reasons for this? During the Renaissance all this changed. Artists began looking at real people before they started painting or carving. It was not good enough just to look at the outside of people's bodies. A lot of artists started to wonder about what was happening under the skin. They wanted to find out about muscles and bones. How could they do this? They did not have X-rays or cameras. To find out about the inside of a person's body they had to learn anatomy. This is what a lot of artists during the Renaissance wanted to do.

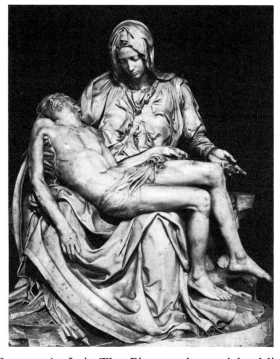

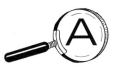

Look at Source A
? What do these statues tell us about Michelangelo's knowledge of bodies?
? How long do you think a statue like the Pieta took him to make?

Look at Source A. It is The Pieta sculptured by Michelangelo Buonarotti. Look at the figures. They are very life-like. Michelangelo's work was all like this. He found out how people's bodies were made, by dissection. What is dissection?

Michelangelo was breaking the law when he dissected bodies. He had to creep into the morgue or a local monastery every night to see if there were any fresh corpses for him to cut up. He was alone in the dark. He was surrounded by decaying corpses. He cut up the bodies to find out about the inside of them. How do you think he might have felt? Do you think he might have learned much?

Source B is from 'The Agony and the Ecstacy' by Irving Stone. The book tells the story of Michelangelo's life. Source B is about his lonely dissections.

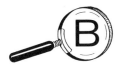

Look at Source B
? What did Michelangelo find out?
? Do you think he was frightened?
? Did he find the job revolting?
? Why did he do it?

Source B
'He made his incisions expertly now, put his hand under the chest bone. It came away easily. Up towards the neck he felt a tube-like appendage, about an inch in diameter that gave the impression of a series of hard rings; among these rings he found a soft tube that came down from the neck. He could not find where this tube ended and the lung began, but when he pulled on it the boys neck and mouth moved. He took his hand out swiftly and shuddered away from the table.'

Another artist who discovered new knowledge from dissection was Leonardo da Vinci. Source C is one of his sketches of the human heart.

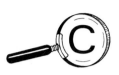

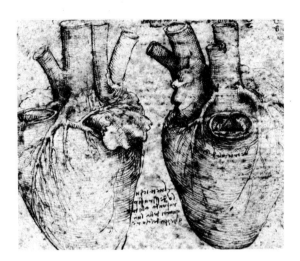

Look at Source C
? What do these sketches show?
? How would Leonardo have found out what a human heart looked like?
? Do you think he might have got into trouble?

Leonardo da Vinci designed a helicopter, a submarine and a tank as well. Why do you think no-one took up his ideas during the Renaissance? Why did we have to wait until the 20th century to see all of these things in use?

Knowledge based on observation

So during the Renaissance artists began studying dead bodies. Did they find out very much?

You only have to look at the statues and paintings done at that time to see what they had learned. They knew all about the bones in the human skeleton. They understood muscles and how they moved. They had become familiar with the insides of bodies.

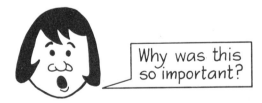

Why was this so important?

Because other people learned about this and used the ideas. Scientists and doctors began to look carefully at things. They stopped guessing and started observing. But they still relied on guidance from the Church and the stars!

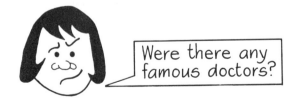

Were there any famous doctors?

Yes. One famous doctor was Andreas Vesalius. You can see his portrait in Source D. Vesalius was very interested in the dissecting being done by artists. As a student doctor he joined artists in the mortuaries to dissect corpses. He was interested in anatomy. Do you think he would have had a lot of real knowledge?

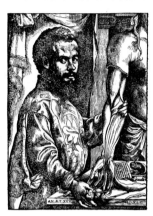

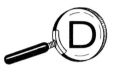

Look at Source D
? What does this show?
? What does it tell us about Vesalius?

Old ideas are destroyed . . . or are they?

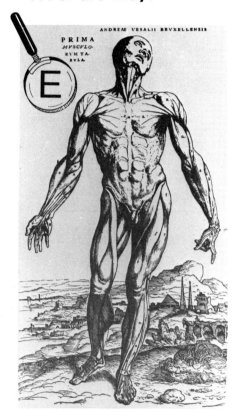

Source E is from a book written by Vesalius. He ordered the building of a dissecting theatre. A lot of students could go there to watch bodies being dissected. That way student doctors found out about the inside of a body.

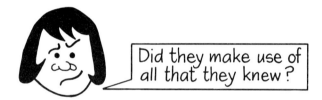

Did they make use of all that they knew?

Sometimes. But many people clung to the old ideas even when they were proved to be wrong. One surgeon tried hard to break away from old ideas and methods. Unfortunately many things still went on as before. The surgeon was called Ambroise Paré. He was a military surgeon. He was always busy. Why do you think Paré was always busy? Ambroise Paré was a clever man. He saw what was wrong with surgery. He tried to correct it. He was a barber-surgeon. He tried to improve medical treatment. He was attempting sensible cures. He also tried to cause less pain to his patients. Source F is from Paré's records.

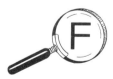

Look at Source F
? Why do you think Paré had not seen gunshot wounds before?
? What was cauterising?
? Why did Paré have to try another cure? What did he use?
? Why do you think he had a sleepless night?
? What was the result of his treatment? Do you think he learned anything from his experience?

Source F

'I had not yet seen wounds made by gunshot . . . For their cure (other doctors command) to cauterise them with oil of elder, scalding hot . . . Eventually my oil lacked and I was constrained to apply in its place a digestive made of the yolks of eggs, oil of roses and turpentine. That night I could not sleep, fearing my lack of cauterisation that I should find the wounded dead or poisoned . . . Beyond my hope I found (them) feeling little pain and . . . inflammation. The others I found feverish with great pain and swelling in their wounds.'

Paré wrote a book called 'Works on Surgery' in 1575. In this book he described amputation. He showed how to cut off a limb. He used a tight strap round the limb. This did three things. It held back muscles and flesh. It stopped the bleeding. It helped to stop the pain. Why were all of these things important? He said that ordinary bandages should be used after the operation. He was not in favour of cauterising the wound. Why?

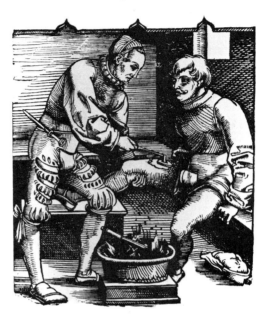

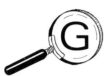

Look at Source G
? What is happening in the picture?
? What does the cautery iron look like? Draw a picture of it.
? Do you think this is a picture of Paré treating a patient?
? Why didn't all surgeons follow his example?

Important discoveries ... were they used?

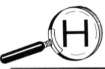

We've seen Vesalius improving anatomy. We've looked at Paré and what he did for surgery. Was there anyone else?

Yes. There was a man called William Harvey. Source H is his portrait.

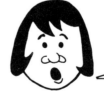

That sounds like an English name.

He was born in England. He became a doctor. He worked for two English kings, James I and Charles I. At first he believed in the ideas of Aristotle, Hippocrates and Galen. Can you remember what these ideas were? Revise them if you cannot. When Harvey dissected frogs he realised that the heart was a pump. It pumped blood around the body. The blood then came back to the heart and to the lungs to get more oxygen. William Harvey had discovered the circulatory system. Source I is an extract from Harvey's diary. He was worried about what other doctors might say about his discovery.

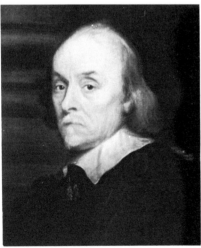

Look at Source I
? Why do you think he was so frightened of suffering their 'ill-will'?
? Which people might have turned against him?
? Why were they afraid of change?

Source I
'I fear that I may not only suffer from the ill will of a few, but dread that all men will turn against me.'

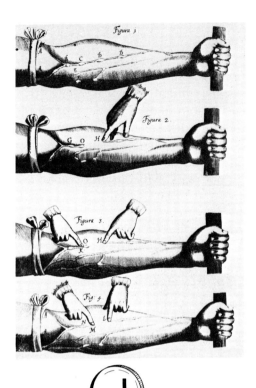

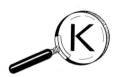

Source J shows illustrations from Harvey's book, of the heart and the actions of the valves in the veins. If the upper arm is bandaged to restrict the flow of blood the valves show up as nodes on the swollen vein. If a finger is pressed along a vein from one valve to the next in a direction away from the heart the section of the vein will be emptied of blood. It will remain empty because the valve does not allow blood to flow away from the heart.

It looks as though the Renaissance was a time when some really clever ideas were started. This looks like real PROGRESS.

That's right. There were new ideas as Source K shows. Doctors tried sensible cures. Looking at patients carefully became very important. But some doctors still tried to cling to stupid and old-fashioned ideas.

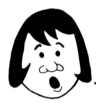

Oh no! Go on then. Tell me some of them.

Source K. Look at this chart. Try to fill in the spaces.

Name	Old way	Changes and new ideas	Effects	Evidence
Michaelangelo Buonorotti				
Versalius	Galen's idea about anatomy			
		New methods of treating gun shot wounds. New ways of amputating limbs.		Works on surgery
	Aristotle's four humours theory. Galen's idea of a vital spirit carried round the body.			Lecture notes and diagrams

Old ideas continue

In Persia there was a type of goat with a hard lump in its stomach. People called this lump the bezoar stone. It was supposed to have magic powers. It was thought to stop poison from hurting people. Crooks used this idea to sell bezoar stone and charge a lot of money for it. Paré tested bezoar on a criminal who was going to be executed, promising him his freedom if the bezoar worked. He gave him poison. He then gave him a drink made from bezoar. The criminal died twelve hours later in terrible pain. Paré had persuaded a lot of people that bezoar did not work but it was still used. If people could see it did not work, why did they still believe in it?

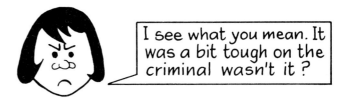

I see what you mean. It was a bit tough on the criminal wasn't it?

Yes. We might not have learned as much as we know today if people had not been brave and experimented. You will see a lot of this in the next units. Try to decide for yourself whether it is worth doing experiments . . . on people or animals.

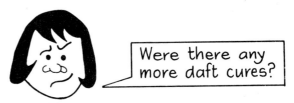

Were there any more daft cures?

Plenty. When Charles II died in February 1685 his doctors had tortured him for five days.

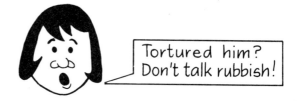

Tortured him? Don't talk rubbish!

OK. Listen to what they did and judge for yourself.

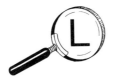

Source L
2nd February 1685.   8 oz blood were taken. An emetic was given to make him sick. Laxatives and an enema were given so that he would have diarrhoea. His head was shaved. Hot blistering poultices were applied.
3rd February.   10 oz blood taken. Gargle with elm bark. More laxatives.
4th February.   More laxatives. Medicine made of spirit of human skull.
5th February.   Peruvian bark medicine given. Very bitter and unpleasant to drink.
6th February.   Bezoar given.

Look at Source L
? Why do you think these treatments were tried?
? Why was King Charles so exhausted?

But alas, after an ill-fated night His Majesty's strength seemed exhausted . . . he expired soon after noon.

62

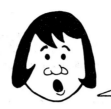

I'm not surprised. Poor King Charles II. Couldn't his doctors see they were doing him more harm than good?

During the Renaissance there was a lot of progress. Doctors learned a lot about anatomy. Surgery got much better. Harvey discovered the circulation of the blood.

At the same time old ideas continued. Old and useless treatments were still used. Doctors used the stars to guide them in the way they treated patients.

Source M shows two of King Charles' doctors. They ordered the strange and cruel treatments for him. You could say that doctors took two steps forward and one step backward.

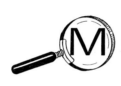

Look at Source M
? Why is this picture such a contradiction of their old ideas?

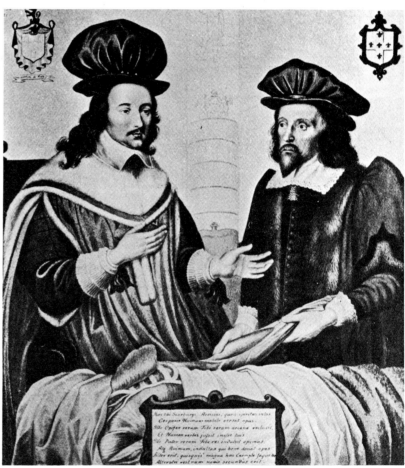

Science improves

Key ideas

New scientific knowledge and ideas.

Changes and improvements.

Identifying progress, even in the process of experimentation.

Discoveries

Medicine today is very advanced. This is because today we know a lot about science and chemistry. Can you think of one instrument that made much of this knowledge possible? Some things are too small to see. Air is usually invisible but it has a lot of things floating in it. A man called Malpighi invented a microscope in about 1680. It was not very good, but it was good enough to show tiny blood capilliaries in the body. This was a very important change. For instance it confirmed Harvey's theory of blood circulation by showing the tiny capilliaries all over the body.

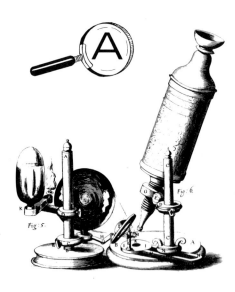

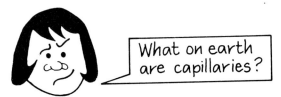

What on earth are capillaries?

Finding out what was wrong with a patient — diagnosis

Very tiny tubes much smaller than veins and arteries. You cannot see them without a microscope. Another man from Holland improved this microscope in 1683. His name was Leeuwenhook. He made the microscope more powerful. You can see this microscope in Source A. He could see things that were so small they were invisible. He was the first person to see bacteria and sperm. This was very important. Can you think of any reasons why? Soon people realised that it might be bacteria that caused illness. Once they had this idea they could start to fight illness.

Pulse

Today it is usual for a doctor or nurse to put their fingers on a sick person's wrist and look at their watch at the same time. What are they doing? What is it called?

Try this:

1 Sit down. Put your fingers on the inside of your wrist below your thumb. You should be able to feel a jumping movement in your wrist. Get someone to time you for 30 seconds. In that time count how many jumps you can feel. Write in your book the amount of movements for 30 seconds.

2 Now get up. Jog on the spot very fast for one minute. Jump up and down for one minute and pump your hands.

3 Sit down. Feel your wrist straight away. Count the jumping movements for 30 seconds. Do you notice any difference? Record the amount in your book.

To us it seems obvious that taking your pulse shows how quickly your heart is working to pump your blood. Three hundred years ago this was not so obvious. A man called Sir John Floyer invented this method of taking a pulse in about AD 1700 but no one used his idea seriously until AD 1850.

Look at Source B
? What is this instrument?
? What problems might Laennec have had with his invention?
? How was Laennec's invention different from the same instruments today?
? Why was the invention such an important change?

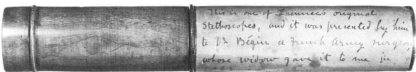

Source B shows an instrument that was invented by a man called Rene Laennec in about AD 1810. A similar instrument is used by doctors today. Laennec's instrument was a roll of paper. He could listen to the noises from his patient's chest through this. Can you think of any ways he could have improved on a roll of paper?

Try this:
With a partner and a roll of paper, place one end against your partner's back or chest and put the other end to your ear. What can you hear? Try to describe the various sounds. How might they help a doctor to decide what was wrong with his patient?

Laennec eventually made a wooden tube. He fixed flexible rubber tubes to it. These went to both ears. He could hear the sounds far more clearly.

Doctors today realise that noises inside a patient's chest can show if there is something wrong with them. In the early 19th century a man called Leo Auenbrugger first used the idea of tapping a patient's chest. He could hear different types of hollow sounds. This helped him to know what was wrong with the patient's chest. This was called auscultation.

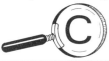

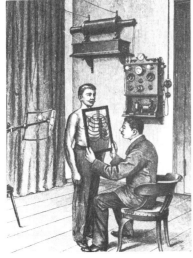

Look at Source C
? Can you think of any ways in which medicine could be helped by X-rays?
? How would it change the treatments doctors gave to their patients?

X-rays

Another important discovery was made in 1896. In Germany, William Röntgen was experimenting with vacuums. He was using a form of photography. He discovered a kind of photography that could show shadows of solid shapes inside a body. This was called X-ray. Suddenly doctors could look inside a body without cutting it open. This helped medicine a lot. Source C shows an early X-ray being taken.

Radium

In France, Pierre and Marie Curie discovered radium. Radium is now used to fight cancer, as well as for other things. It was a very important discovery. It could be used to treat illness but it could also cause illness unless great care was taken. Marie Curie herself died of pernicious anaemia. This is a form of cancer of the blood.

Blood transfusions

Once William Harvey had discovered the circulation of the blood, people began to experiment in transferring blood from animals to patients or from other people to patients. In his diary, Samuel Pepys talks of this. Look at Source D.

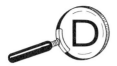

Look at Source D
? What did Pepys think about the experiment?
? What did the experiment show?
? What sort of jokes did they make about it?
? What was it hoped to cure?

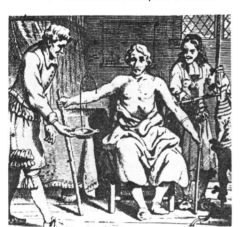

Source D
14th November 1666
'Doctor Croone told me at the meeting of Gresham College tonight . . . there was a pretty experiment of the blood of one dog let out till he died, into the body of another on one side, while all his run out on the other side. The first dies upon the place and the other very well and likely to do well.
'This did give occasion to many pretty wishes, as of the blood of the Quaker to be let into an Archbishop and such like; but, as Dr Croone says, it may if it takes, be of mighty use to a man's health, for the amending of bad blood by borrowing from a better body.'

Pepys was referring to experiments carried out on dogs by Richard Lower. On 12th June 1667, Jean-Baptiste Denis succeeded in giving blood from a lamb to a dying man The man survived. These were lucky chances. We know today that a person can only be given blood of the same group as his own. Karl Landsteiner showed this in 1899.

Today blood transfusions are carried out regularly. Dialysis machines can clean the blood of patients with poor kidneys. Blood banks have been set up by the National Blood Transfusion Service. Donors are called to give blood every six months. This service has saved thousands of lives.

A vast number of changes took place in this era, 1600–1850. Simple scientific ideas like these helped medicine to improve. The invention of microscopes was very important. Doctors were still interested in dissecting dead bodies. These dissections gave a lot of information about the body. It showed diseases and injuries. When doctors had seen these they had better ideas of how to treat them in their own patients. But a lot of dead bodies were needed . . . How could they be found?

Cause and effect of change

Dead bodies were not easy to find. Families wanted their dead relatives buried decently. It was not respectable to have anything to do with dissection.

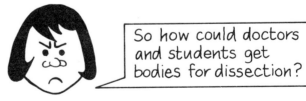

So how could doctors and students get bodies for dissection?

Before 1828, the bodies of criminals who were executed were not given to their relatives.

Look at Source E
? Why did Henry VIII pass a law giving away corpses?
? Why are Barbers and Surgeons mentioned together?

Source E
Henry VIII passed a law giving corpses of criminals to the Company of Barbers and Surgeons.

Resurrection men

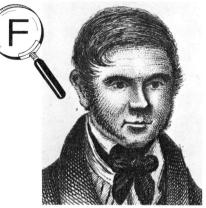

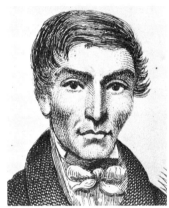

? Burke (top) and Hare (bottom). Being a resurrection man was a very dangerous job. How many reasons can you think of for it being so dangerous?

The interest in anatomy grew. There were not enough bodies. Students had to pay a fee to watch a dissection. Professors who dissected corpses were forced to pay for the bodies. Do you think they were pleased to get the bodies? Why? Dead bodies became big business!

If medicine was to progress, dissection had to be carried out. There were men who made a business out of obtaining dead bodies. They were called Resurrection Men. Why do you think they were given this name? When they heard of a death they would watch the funeral. They would then return to the grave the same night and dig up the body. Why would they rob the grave so quickly? How do you think they would do it?

This body snatching became very common. The prices of bodies went up. Some doctors tried to form a club to get bodies for themselves. The professional body snatchers did not like this. They started dumping very old corpses on doctors' doorsteps. Why did they do this?

In 1828 body snatching reached its revolting climax. In Edinburgh, William Burke and William Hare supplied Dr Knox with corpses. You can see Burke and Hare in Source F. When there were no fresh corpses they murdered people to provide fresh bodies. They were caught by the police. Burke was executed. Hare gave evidence against him. This was called 'Turning King's Evidence'. He was released but a mob murdered him and threw his body in a lime pit. Why do you think the mob were so cruel to William Hare?

In London, John Bishop and James May were doing the same sorts of things as Burke and Hare. They were caught when they tried to sell a dentist some teeth from one of their victims. Unfortunately they forgot to take the gums off!

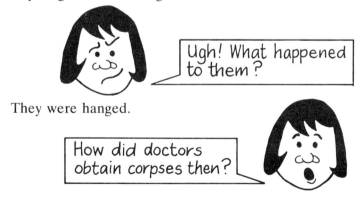

Ugh! What happened to them?

They were hanged.

How did doctors obtain corpses then?

The British Government passed an Act in 1832. It was called the Anatomy Act. Leaving bodies to medical science was up to either the relatives or the people themselves.

This Act shows that the medical profession still needed bodies for dissection. It still does today. The Government, because of pressure from the medical profession, made it legal to donate dead bodies for dissection. Today a lot of people carry donor cards. These allow doctors to take organs from their bodies if they are killed in an accident.

List the changes we have seen in medicine in this Unit. What effects did they have?

Dissection?

? Why is there a need for bodies for dissection today?
? Try to obtain a donor card. Draw a picture of it in your book. Why does it mention certain organs? Are they to be dissected?

Fighting disease

Key ideas

Use of experiment based on guesswork.

Use of experiment based on knowledge.

Causes of disease

The means of fighting bacteria and germs.

Vaccination

The cartoon in Source A was drawn in 1802 by a man called Gilray.

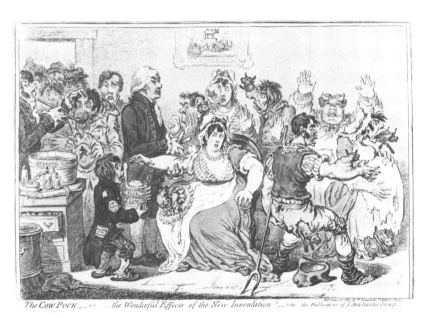

The COW POCK ___ ___ the Wonderful Effects of the New Inoculation ! ___ vide. the Publications of ᵞ Anti Vaccine Society

Look at Source A
? What is the man standing in the middle of the cartoon doing?
? Who is his patient? Does the patient look pleased? Why?
? What unusual things are happening to other people in the cartoon?
? Look at the picture on the back wall. What is happening? Why do you think that picture is there?

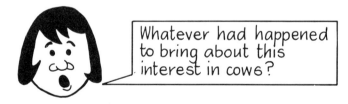

Whatever had happened to bring about this interest in cows?

In 1796, a man called Edward Jenner was a doctor in a Gloucestershire village. His patients often died of smallpox. Smallpox was a dangerous disease. There was no way to cure it then. Jenner realised that dairymaids did not get smallpox but they did catch cowpox from their cows. This was similar to smallpox but not as dangerous. Jenner believed that catching cowpox protected people against smallpox. How do you think he arrived at this conclusion?

He was not exactly sure why cowpox gave protection against smallpox but had some ideas. To find if his ideas were right, he experimented on a small boy.

Jenner's experiment

He cut the boy's arm. He put some matter from a cowpox blister into the cut. The boy caught cowpox. Later he did the same thing but this time he used matter from a smallpox blister. The boy was all right. He was protected. His own body had fought off the smallpox. This was called **vaccination**, a word that comes from the Latin word for cow. Edward Jenner didn't understand why vaccination worked. He had not seen the bacteria that caused smallpox because microscopes that could magnify that much were not then available, but he had made a big step forward.

In the 1800s doctors began to realise that germs and bacteria caused disease but there was no **proof**.

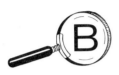

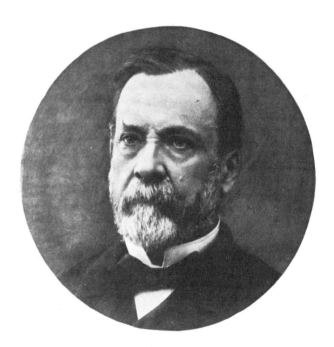

Source B shows Louis Pasteur. He was not a doctor, he was a chemist. He lived in France. A wine merchant was having trouble with wine turning sour. He asked Pasteur to help him. Pasteur realised that germs were causing the wine to go sour. The germs in the air were the cause of the disease. Source C is from a lecture that Pasteur gave in 1864.

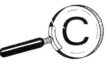

Look at Source C
? How did Pasteur destroy the germs in the liquid?
? How did the liquid get contaminated again?
? What did this prove?

Source C
'By boiling, I destroyed any germs contained in the liquid or against the glass; but that liquid being again in contact with the air, it became altered.'

Microbe hunting

Pasteur discovered that illness was caused by germs. It was carried through the air. He tried to show that this was how wounds and surgical operations became infected. But he still could not identify the germs that caused certain illnesses. What had Pasteur discovered about germs? We still have pasteurised milk today. Why do you think it is given this name?

Source D shows Robert Koch. He was a German scientist. He worked for many years to find out about microbes that caused disease.

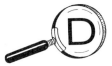

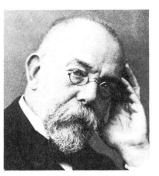

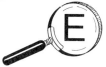

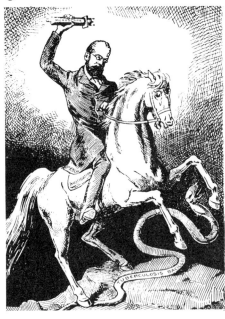

Look at Source E
? Why is Koch shown as St. George?
? What is his dragon? Was he successful in fighting it?

They are bacteria. They cause disease. Microbes are so small that they are virtually invisible. How do you think Koch studied microbes if they were invisible to the human eye?

Koch learnt a lot about anthrax germs. Anthrax was a fatal animal disease. People could catch it too. Koch discovered that anthrax germs made spores that survived for a long time.

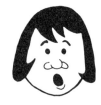

They are like tiny eggs. They grow into germs. Koch had discovered that germs breed and multiply. Bacteriology or Microbe-hunting became very popular. A lot of progress was made. Progress is still being made. Can you think of any disease today that scientists are still trying to learn about?

Yes. The main thing he did was studying the germs that caused septicaemia.

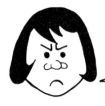

70

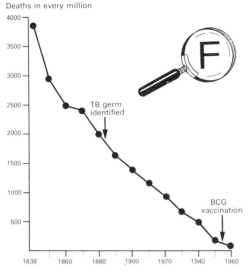

Deaths in every million

TB germ identified

BCG vaccination

Septicaemia is blood poisoning. It is usually caused by infection of open wounds in someone's body. It often occurs if wounds are not cleaned properly. In 1880 Koch at last discovered the germ that causes tuberculosis or TB. This is a terrible disease. One hundred years ago many people died from TB. Koch's discoveries meant that these diseases could be fought. It had taken a long time. Vaccines were developed. Many of them were found by chance or long experimentation.

Look at Source F
? Why did so many people die of TB in 1838?
? Why did the number of deaths drop after 1880?
? Why are there so few deaths from TB today?

Chemotherapy

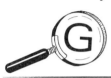

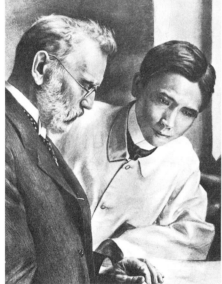

People had learned a lot about the germs that caused disease. Doctors could prevent some diseases by using vaccines but they often could not cure disease. Doctors needed something that would kill the germs without killing the patient. Source G shows two men who worked very hard on this problem. They are Paul Ehrlich and Sahachiro Hata.

These two men developed Salvarsan 606. This chemical was injected into a patient. It would kill all the germs it came across. Salvarsan was very successful. It began a new age. **The age of chemotherapy.**

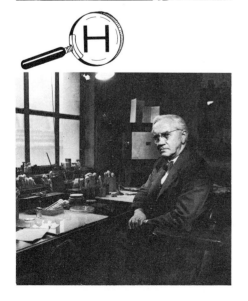

Diseases were fought with chemicals called drugs. The most useful discovery was a drug called penicillin. This is still used today. A doctor called Alexander Fleming had seen soldiers in World War I die of blood poisoning. Their wounds were deep and badly infected. He wanted to discover a drug to prevent this terrible suffering. You can see Fleming at work in Source H. What he actually discovered was a kind of mould. An extract of this mould could destory a lot of different germs. It was turned into a medicine by Howard Florey and Ernst Chain and was first tried out in mice. What was the reason for this? Eventually, in 1940, penicillin was used on a policeman with blood poisoning. The man recovered. Penicillin worked. (The drug ran out and the man died later.) When and where do you think it was first used on a lot of people?

Diseases still spread today. Cancer is a major killer. AIDS has become a household fear. Might a cure be found . . . by chance or by experimentation?

Better surgery

Key ideas

Two problems of surgery — pain and infection.

Causes and effects of these problems.

Improvements achieved by individuals.

Problems

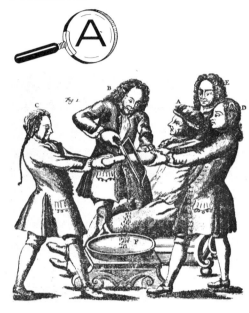

As we have seen, Ambroise Paré had already made some improvement in surgical operations. By 1800 there was still a long way to go. There were two main problems that had to be solved. Can you think what these problems were? Source A should give you some clues.

Look at Source A
? Who is operating on the patient? How is he dressed?
? What tools and instruments is he using?
? What operation is he doing?
? What is happening to the patient?
? Who are the other people? What are they doing?

The two main problems of surgery were:
1 There was terrible pain during the operation.
2 There was a serious risk of infection or bleeding to death.
Doctors had to solve these problems.
Let's look at pain first.

Early methods of pain relief

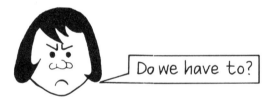

Do we have to?

Yes. Pain is unpleasant. It can cause shock and even death. Surgeons needed to find a way to stop the patient feeling pain during the operation. If they did this, longer and more careful operations could be carried out.

We have seen that operations have been carried out for thousands of years. Do you remember the trephining operation in Unit 1? How do you think Stone Age people dealt with the problem of pain?

Doctors had tried several ways of dealing with pain.

1 Knocking a patient out was usual. Why was this a bad idea?

2 Some herbs were used. There were things like lettuce leaves and opium from poppies. Why do you think these were not very successful?

3 **Alcohol** was often used. This might have been more pleasant. Can you list any difficulties in using alcohol to stop pain?

4 When everything else failed people were tied up. Can you imagine the fear and agony that a patient would go through?

Something far better was needed. Something far better was found. **Anaesthetics were discovered.**

I remember what anaesthetics are! They are pain killers that put you to sleep but don't permanently harm.

That's right. The discovery of anaesthetics started in about 1800.

1 Sir Humphrey Davy used **nitrous oxide** to kill the pain of toothache. He called nitrous oxide 'laughing gas' because it made people very giggly and silly! By 1840 other doctors were using it. It was not always a success. An American dentist called Horace Wells was booed out of the room where he was demonstrating nitrous oxide to an audience. This was because his patient moaned loudly when Wells took his tooth out. His audience of students shouted that his discovery was 'humbug' — in other words **Rubbish!** Why were people so unwilling to believe in Well's demonstration of laughing gas?

2 In 1846 surgeons tried **ether** on their patients. A famous surgeon called Robert Liston used it very successfully on his patients. He carried out amputations using ether to stop his patients' pain. In Source B he is operating on a man who is suffering no pain.

Look at Source B
? Where is the ether spray? Try drawing it in your book.
? Is there anything wrong with the operation? Pain has been lessened but what problems are still there?

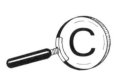

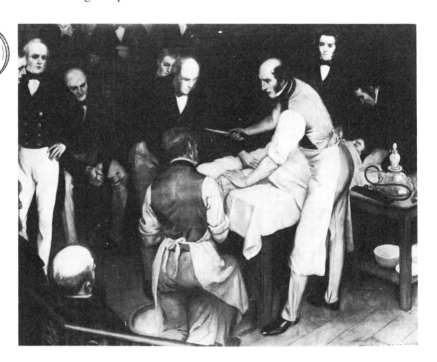

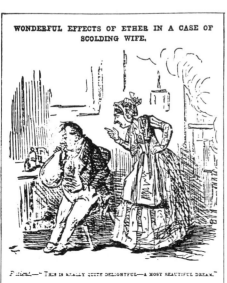

WONDERFUL EFFECTS OF ETHER IN A CASE OF SCOLDING WIFE.

Patient.—" THIS IS REALLY QUITE DELIGHTFUL—A MOST BEAUTIFUL DREAM."

Michael Faraday took ether to fairgrounds. He set up tents for 'ether frolics'. What do you think these might have been? Source C shows another use of ether. It was a good anaesthetic but it could be dangerous if it was carelessly used. Some patients died from using ether.

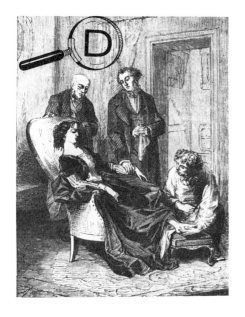

3 James Simpson was a young professor of midwifery at Edinburgh University. He and some friends experimented with **chloroform.** They all became unconscious — they had discovered a new anaesthetic. It became popular when Queen Victoria was given it at the birth of two of her children. It could be dangerous. There were some deaths from the use of chloroform. Source D shows the first death. The patient's name was Hannah Green. There were risks but they were worth it.

The individual people who believed in their discoveries had the courage to carry on with their work. Many people benefited because of this. Source E shows a letter from John Churchill, a patient of Robert Liston.

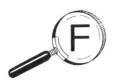

Look at Source E
? What does this letter tell us about the opinons of ordinary people about surgery?
? What does John Churchill think about anaesthetics?

Source E

'Several years ago I was required to prepare for the loss of a limb by amputation. Suffering so great as I underwent cannot be expressed in words. I still recall the spreading out of the instruments, the first incision and the bloody limb lying on the floor. From all this I should have been saved by ether or chloroform.'

Anaesthetics today

Today we have a lot of different anaesthetics. Different painkillers are used for different things. Some of these are shown in Source F.

Table F. Different kinds of anaesthetic.

Kind of anaesthetic	Use
Local anaesthetic, which is often made from cocaine.	Stitching wounds Cleaning wounds Having teeth out.
Barbiturate anaesthetic, which is usually injected. This very quickly puts you to sleep.	For making patients unconscious for surgical operations
Sedatives, which can take several forms — injections, tablets and breathing entynox gas.	Makes a patient drowsy Makes a patient care less about pain (These are often used in childbirth)
Epidural anaesthetic, this is local anaesthetic injected into the spine. It dulls nerve endings and cuts off pain.	It is used in childbirth and for artificial joint replacements in old people
TENS is a new anaesthetic. This is electric current used to dull nerve endings	It is used in childbirth

Try to find out anything you can about any of these. See if you can find someone who has been given one of these anaesthetics. Ask them what it was like. Record their answers.

Infection

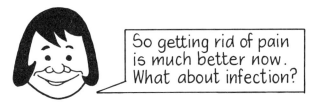

So getting rid of pain is much better now. What about infection?

This problem was a serious one. Infection was caused by germs. These were in the room where the operation took place. The germs were in clothing, on furniture, on people. Germs were everywhere even if they were not recognised.

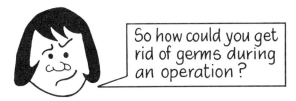

So how could you get rid of germs during an operation?

Many surgeons were good people. They cared about their patients. But very often it was the surgeons who killed the patients. They wore their ordinary clothes during the operation. Surgery took place in an ordinary room. Surgeons often invited an audience to watch them. They didn't often wash their hands before surgery. The surgeons even carried their suture thread wrapped round their buttons!

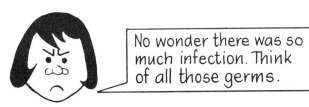

No wonder there was so much infection. Think of all those germs.

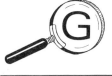

Pasteur and Koch had shown that germs caused disease. Surgeons tried to use this knowledge. Source G shows Joseph Lister. He realised that germs in the operating theatre had to be destroyed. Lister used **carbolic acid spray** in the operating room. This was to kill the germs. It was very successful. He insisted that all doctors and nurses should wash their hands in carbolic before touching a patient. This was not very popular. Why was the use of carbolic so unpopular? Lister even used carbolic acid for dressing wounds. It soon became clear that his patients did not get infected. Carbolic acid was one of the first **antiseptics**. It killed germs in wounds. It also killed germs in the air and in the operating room. Source H shows the carbolic spray.

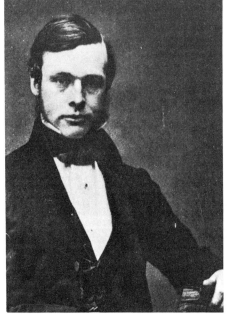

Look at Source H.
? What does the spray look like?
? In what other ways could Lister have improved the operating room?

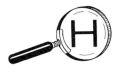

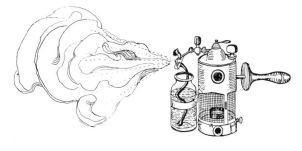

Other people worked hard to fight infection in operating theatres and hospitals. In 1847, a doctor in Hungary called Albert Semmelweis was very worried about puerperal fever. This was an infection after childbirth that killed a lot of mothers. Semmelweis saw doctors and students dissecting bodies. The same people then went to the maternity wards to examine new mothers. Many mothers died from the infection that was unwittingly passed on to them. Semmelweis insisted on all doctors washing their hands in calcium chloride before examining new mothers. The number of deaths fell very quickly. Like Lister, Semmelweis was very unpopular with other doctors. Why do you think this was?

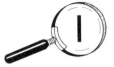

There were a lot of improvements. Look at Source I. It shows some of the improvements. Try to fill in the improvements showing who was involved and what results each improvement might have.

Table I. Development of antiseptic surgery.

Improvement	Result
Using an old coat for operating in was stopped	
The 'ward sponge' was not used any more. This had been used for every kind of dressing and cleaning.	
1890 — Surgeons now used rubber gloves	
1900 — Caps, masks and gowns were used by surgeons and their assistants	
Surgical instruments were sterilised by steam	

Source J shows how far modern surgery has developed. This is the Charnley–Howorth Surgicair operating enclosure. It provides an almost totally sterile atmosphere, although it is now not often used.

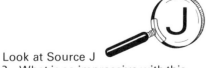

Look at Source J
? What is so impressive with this development?
? What are the differences between this scene and that in Source A.
? Explain in your own words how this operating theatre works.

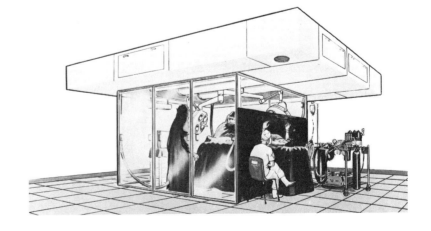

Modern surgery

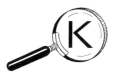

Modern surgery makes use of all the discoveries we have seen. Pain during operations has been stopped. Pain after operations is dealt with by using pain-killing drugs. Risk of infection is lowered by using sterile operating theatres, gowns, instruments and equipment.

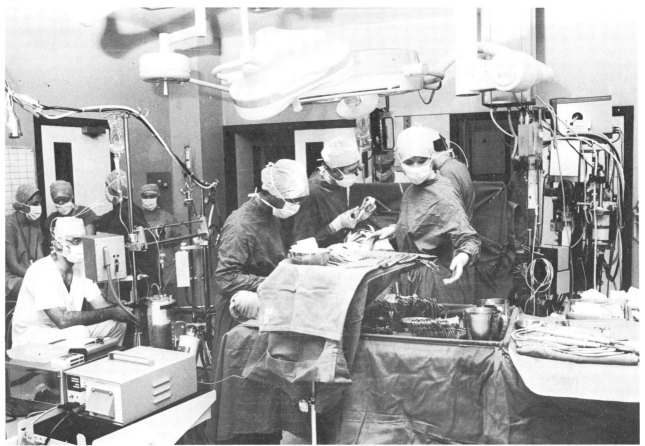

Look at Source K
? What other things are being used to improve a patient's chance of recovery?

Modern surgery involves electrical equipment and monitors. It needs very advanced scientific methods of treatment. Many individuals are working all the time to make modern surgery more impressive. In the 1960s, Professor Christiaan Barnard performed the first heart transplants in humans. Now heart and lung transplants are a fairly routine, though complicated, event. In Britain teams of surgeons at Papworth Hospital and Harefield Hospital do these transplants regularly.

Skin grafting for burns and similar injuries has developed rapidly. The high-powered violence of our world today — bombs, nuclear accidents, advanced weapons — have all had effects on surgery. Surgery has developed to cope with these problems. Brain surgery is commonplace. Humans can be kept alive with the aid of modern technology.

But every advance was made by individuals. Every operation still relies on the skill of the individual surgeon.

Hospitals and nursing

Key ideas

The idea of hospitals has changed little.

Many methods, techniques and situations continue.

Changes are often developments of ideas thousands of years old.

Early hospitals

Can you remember all about the dream houses in Ancient Egypt? Think back to the healing temple where sick people went to get help from Asclepios. These places had wards with a number of beds in them. There were people to look after the patients. The diet was fairly good. The patients enjoyed fresh air and exercise. Dream houses and healing temples were a bit like hospitals. They were also health resorts and convalescent homes. Try drawing a cartoon strip to show all these things.

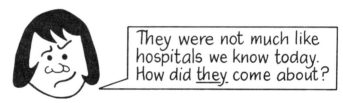

They were not much like hospitals we know today. How did <u>they</u> come about?

Roman military hospitals were like our hospitals today. In Roman times there were some small hospitals for poor people. These were usually set up in the homes of rich, upper-class ladies. One of these was called Fabiola. She set up a charity hospital in Sabina in AD 400. Why do you think rich, upper-class ladies spent their time founding hospitals?

This idea carried on even after the Roman Empire collapsed. France had a lot of hospitals. A lot of these were started by rich ladies. The ladies were sometimes very religious. They dedicated the hospitals to God.

Princess Margaret of Burgundy founded a hospital in 1293. It was built at Tonnere in France. A lot of records were kept about the building. Diaries were kept by some of the people who worked there. All of these documents give us an idea of what the hospital was like. Look at Source A.

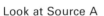

Look at Source A
? List the ways in which this hospital is different from hospitals today?
? What things are the same?
? Why do you think ventilation was important?
? Do you think it might have been a good hospital? Why?

Source A

'It was isolated. The ward was 18½ metres wide and 90 metres long. There was good ventilation and all the cubicles were tiled. Colourful stained glass was in the windows. There was drainage and a water supply by means of a stream.'

Other hospitals were as good as this. St Thomas's Hospital was founded in London in AD 1215. It was another charity hospital. Arab doctors were working in organised hospitals. A proper hospital was built in Damascus in AD 1160. It gave free medical treatment to everyone.

But most hospitals in the Middle Ages were very poor. They were badly built. There was no ventilation or heating. Doctors and nurses didn't know much about hygiene. Patients shared beds, food and equipment. A lot of people died in these hospitals.

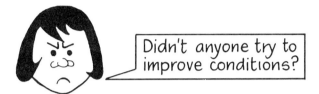

Didn't anyone try to improve conditions?

Yes. Monks and nuns worked hard to make things easier for those who were ill. Most monasteries had infirmaries. In the infirmaries trained monks and nuns looked after sick people.

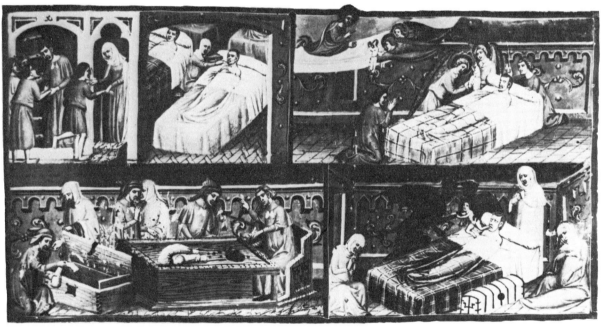

Look at Source B
? List all of the things that show they didn't know much about hygiene?
? What examples are there of good nursing skills?
? Does the picture show anything that happens in hospitals today? List these.

The nuns in Source B are attempting good medical treatment. They are both dedicated and skilled. Many nurses from 1600 to 1900 were nothing like this. In his book 'Pickwick Papers', Charles Dickens writes about Sarey Gamp. She was a midwife and nurse. She was dirty, bedraggled and usually drunk. Alcohol was the main treatment she pressed on her patients. Nurses in general had a bad reputation. There must have been some good nurses but the majority were not well liked!

Nursing and hospitals improve

In the 1700s there was a group of people called Quakers. They were very religious. They believed that they should work hard for God. One of these Quakers was Thomas Guy. He founded Guy's Hospital in London. This was well organised and the nurses were fairly well trained. There was also a famous Quaker hospital in York. It was called 'The Retreat'. Its founder was William Tuke. He believed that people who were mentally ill were badly treated.

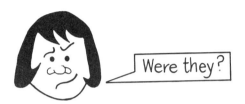

Were they?

Yes. The insane had always been chained up. Treatments were horrible — things like boiling baths and freezing showers. People paid to go and watch lunatics in their cages. One famous hospital in London was called Bedlam. How do we use the word 'bedlam' today?

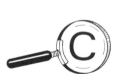

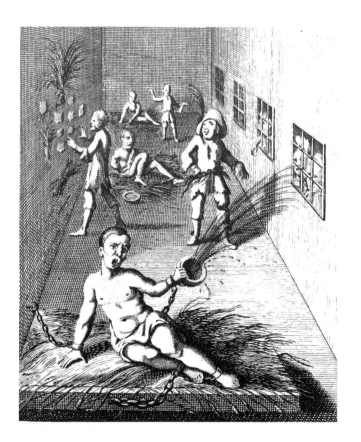

Look at Source C
? How does it show mental patients?
? Do we still have strange ideas about mental illness today?
? What sort of skills would nurses need if they worked with the insane?

Places like 'The Retreat' and Guy's Hospital made nursing more respectable. Patients who were mentally ill received far better treatment. Certain standards were set for nurses. They were expected to try to help their patients.

As well as hospitals there were Medical Missions. These were often run by the Church. Sometimes they were organised by the Salvation Army. Source D is called Prayers before Pills.

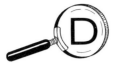

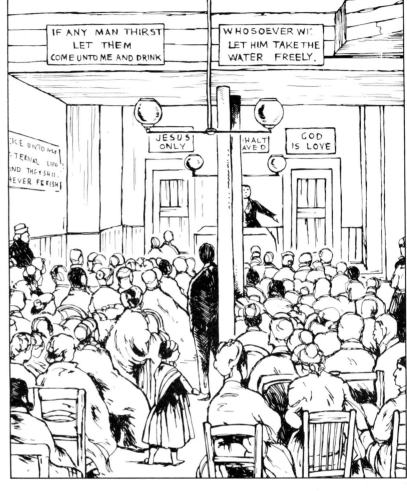

Look at Source D
? Why do you think it has the title 'Prayers before Pills'?
? Do you think medical missions were popular?
? What sort of people might have gone there?
? Is there any continuity between monasteries and these missions?

Source E shows how far hospitals had improved by 1890. Each patient occupied his own bed. Wards were clean. Nurses were smart and tidy. Doctors visited the wards.

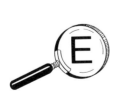

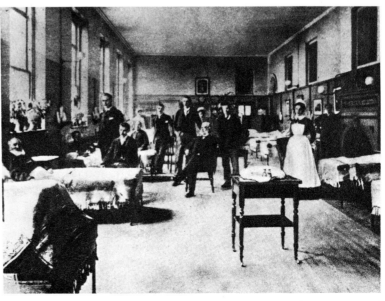

Look at Source E
? List the differences between this and Source B.
? Joseph Lister is in this picture. Has the hospital used any of his ideas about hygiene?
? Is it like a modern hospital as you know it?

81

Florence Nightingale

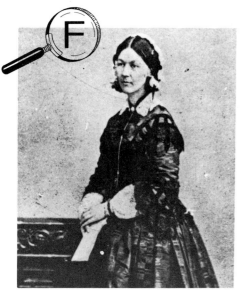

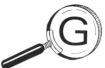

Things were getting better but there was still improvement to be made. Patients still often died. Doctors could not always give the treatment and care that was needed. Look at Source G. It was this lady who helped to make hospitals and nursing as good as they are today. Her name was Florence Nightingale. Her parents were rich. They didn't want her to be a nurse as it was not a very respectable job. Florence Nightingale was determined. She believed God had called her to work with the sick.

She trained in Germany and France and worked voluntarily in charity hospitals and workhouses. She worked with the poor. She saw things she didn't like. What sort of things might she have seen that she disapproved of? Eventually she became superintendent at a home for sick gentlewomen. She introduced into hospitals all kinds of new ideas. These included bells for patients to call nurses and lifts to help nurses move patients.

At this time Britain was involved in fighting in the Crimean War. In 1854, Florence Nightingale was asked to recruit 40 nurses and go to the Crimea. Conditions were terrible. There were no toilets. There was no water or food. Wounded men were lying crammed together with no treatment. More were dying of disease than of their wounds.

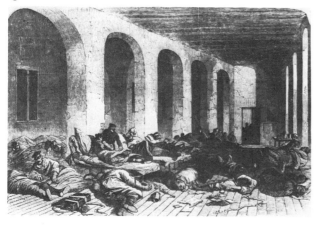 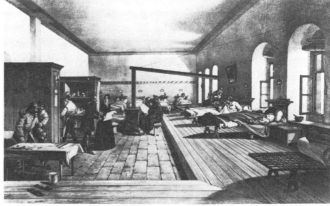

Look at Source G left and right.
? What sort of problems might Florence Nightingale and her nurses have had to face when they arrived in the Crimea?
? What has been done in the right hand picture to improve conditions?

Florence Nightingale fought hard to change the terrible conditions. She was loved and adored. In the end she was very successful. After the war, she came back to London. In 1851 Queen Victoria asked her to set up a college for training nurses, which she did. Hospitals and nursing improved a lot. The State Registered Nurse examination was started by Florence Nightingale. Most nurses today still work to pass this examination.

So far in this book we have seen that most of the famous people improving medicine were men. Florence Nightingale was an exception but women had always been important in nursing and medicine. Women were already doing a lot for medicine in the Middle Ages because they delivered all the babies that were born.

Women were only allowed to train as doctors in Britain after 1860 but were not allowed to qualify until 1876. Today there are about 14,000 women doctors in England. In 1870 there was one. Source H shows Elizabeth Garrett-Anderson. She worked hard to become the first woman doctor trained in Britain, but she had to take her exams in Paris.

People ridiculed her. She didn't have many patients at first. Today women and men doctors are treated the same. They can gain any position if they are qualified. Men are now training as nurses. What do you think about this? Do you think that men will train to become midwives? If so what might they be called? What things are included in nursing skills today?

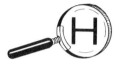

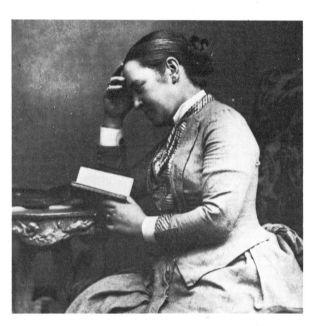

There have been hospitals since very early history. Some aspects of treatment in them have continued. Some have progressed and developed but the basic ideas remain the same.

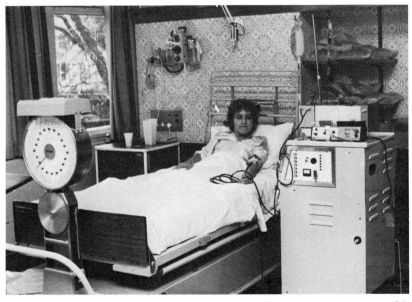

Public health

Key ideas

Public health today.

How public health developed.

The effects of public health measures on all of us.

Major changes in ideas about environment.

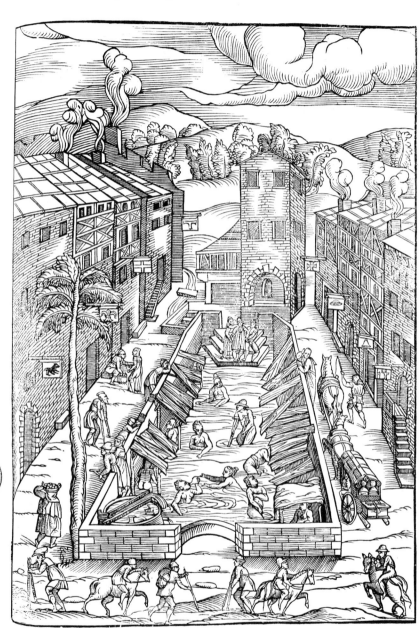

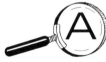

Look at Source A
? Why is this not a satisfying way of keeping clean?
? What improvements would you have made?

Look around you at your town, village or even your school. You can see many ways in which you are protected from illness. List as many of these as you can. We take these protections for granted but they have not always been there.

Looking at the history of medicine tells us a lot of things. One of the main things it shows us is that people have not always understood about germs. They didn't always realise that germs live in dirt. A lot of people have died because of this.

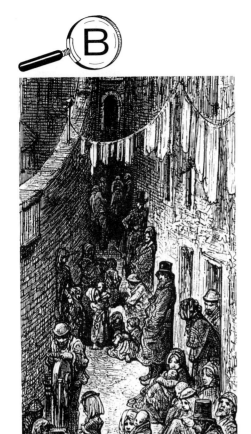

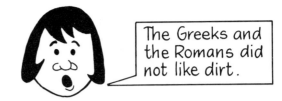

The Greeks and the Romans did not like dirt.

You are right. They washed and they tried to keep their streets, towns and houses clean. Some people in the Middle Ages tried to keep themselves clean. Source A shows a mediaeval bath-house.

As you can see this was not perfect. Many people could not even visit a bath-house. They lived in dirty houses that were often built of unhygienic materials. Often they did not wash. Why was this? Their towns were filthy. Their streets must have smelt terrible. Look at Source B. It shows a street in about 1800. These sorts of conditions existed in some towns until recently. In some places these conditions still exist.

Look at Source B
? List the things that might have been a risk to health?
? Imagine walking down a street like this in 1800. Write about what you saw, the smells and your feelings about it.
? Why do some countries today still have conditions like these?

Source C shows prints of 'Gin Lane' and 'Beer Street'. They were painted by William Hogarth in 1751. Gin was very cheap. It was very strong. The poor people bought a lot of gin. It was their only pleasure. There was a saying, 'Drunk for a penny, dead drunk for twopence'.

Gin was so strong that a lot of people died of alcohol poisoning when they drank it. Mothers were not taught how to look after babies. Sometimes they gave babies bread soaked in gin to keep them quiet. They gave them laudanum too. This was a very strong drug. A lot of people died of the effects of drink. The Government in England put a tax on gin. This made it more expensive so fewer people bought it and fewer people died. This change resulted in improvement in public health.

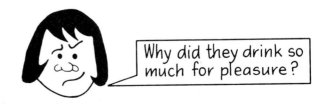

Why did they drink so much for pleasure?

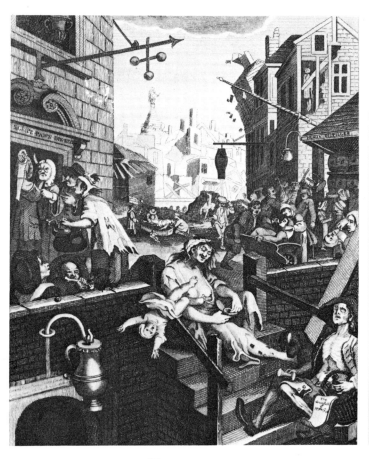
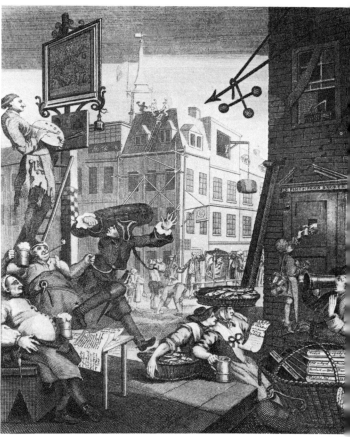

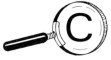

Look at Source C
? Find these things:
  (a) the man who has hanged himself
  (b) the pawn brokers shop
  (c) the woman who is dropping her baby
  Why are all these things happening?
? What is the cause of all this poverty?
? What is there in C that shows what houses like to live in then?
? What improvements does the second picture show? Why?

The people worked long hours. They worked in dirty, noisy factories and mines. Sometimes they worked for 16 hours in every day. Their wages were low. They could not afford much food.

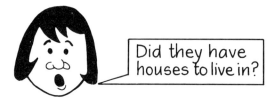

Did they have houses to live in?

Yes. The houses were often built by factory owners or land owners. They were built quickly. Some factory owners spent as little money as they could in building these houses. Why was this? Source D shows a close of houses in Leeds in the 1800s. In industrial towns all over Britain houses like these were built around courtyards. Try to find an example in your area.

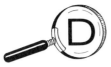

Look at Sources D and E
? How many people do you think lived in each house?
? Did they have toilets and bathrooms?
? Where did they put the rubbish and sewage?
? How do you think they got drinking water?
? What effects would living in these houses have on their health?

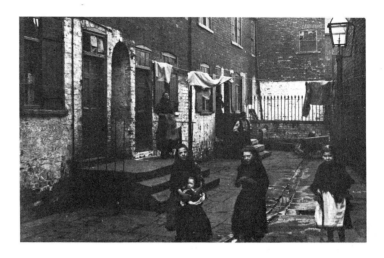

Source E is from a report on the condition of residences of the labouring classes in Leeds in 1842 by R Baker.

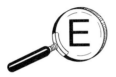

Source E
'Thomas Rooley is 66 years of age. His wife is also about the same age; worked formerly as a soap boiler; is now unable to work and lives on parish allowance, and the earnings of his wife. Has 2s 6d a week . . . Has lived in this cottage for more than twelve month; has had very bad health during that period, and his wife also has had rheumatism. The water in front of the house has accumulated from various sources. The yard has never been dry since he came to it. There is a sump hole, a great depth, in one corner, made by the landlord to take the water away; but it is full of deposit. The stench is often so bad, and especially after rain; that he and his wife cannot bear it.'

Source F shows the average age of people when they died. It shows the difference in the health of people living in the town and those living in the country.

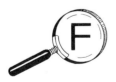

Source F. Average age of death in 1842.
? What does this table tell you about life in the country and in the cities?
? Why are there differences in the average ages of death between people in different jobs?

Source F. Average age of death in 1842.

Type of people	Town	Country
Gentry and their families	44	52
Farmers, tradesmen and their families	27	41
Labourers and their families	19	38

Source G is from an 'Enquiry into the State and Conditions of the Town of Leeds'. It was a government enquiry that was trying to find out how the poor lived. These extracts are from its findings.

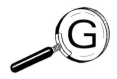

Look at Source G (extracts)
? What other towns might have had the same conditions in 1842?
? Look at your town. Try to find any evidence to show whether or not it had conditions like these in the 1840s.
? How do the extracts in G agree with sources D and E?

Source G

1842 'In one cul-de-sac in Leeds there are 34 houses, and there dwell in these houses 340 people, of ten to every house.'
'One sleeping room must be inadequate for a family of five persons, oftener eight.'
'Neighbourhoods have arisen where there are neither water or offices.'

1834 Leeds water supply

'No water except from wells and rainwater. The water is raised from the river.'
'The sewage is emptied into the river. Privies so laden with ashes and excrement as to be unusable, till the streets themselves were offensive.'

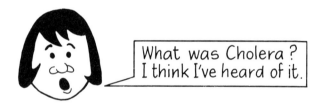

Are you telling me that there were no proper toilets? All the sewage was going straight into the water supply or lying in the streets? That's disgusting! Didn't it cause any major diseases?

Yes. Cholera began in Sunderland in 1831. Can you think of any reasons why it started in Sunderland?

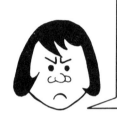

What was Cholera? I think I've heard of it.

Cholera outbreaks

Cholera still exists in parts of the world today. It causes fever, vomiting and diarrhoea. People can die of it very quickly. It spreads very easily and quickly. Cholera started killing thousands of people all over England. It was worst in the large cities. Leeds had a very bad epidemic of cholera in 1831–2. Look at the pictures in source H. These show cholera scenes.

Some people were very worried about bad conditions in towns. They saw that unless things were improved a lot more people would die. Source I shows Edwin Chadwick. He wrote a report on the conditions in Leeds. He made sure the Government saw the report.

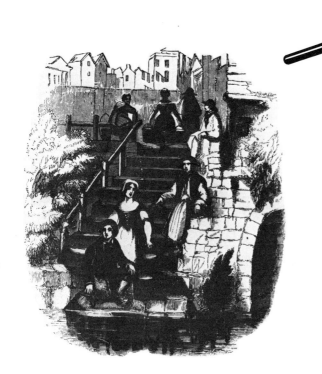

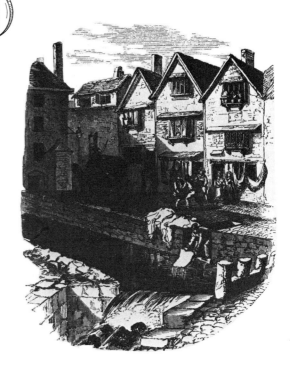

Look at Source H
? What might the authorities in a town try to do about cholera?
? List ways in which cholera could spread.
? List the names of any other diseases that were caused by bad conditions in towns.
? What changes were needed?
? Why is cholera not in Britain today?

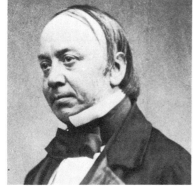

How did they try to improve things?

Changes and improvements

Chadwick and a lot of other people set up local boards of health. These did a lot of good things but they were not popular with the factory owners. Many of the factory owners were wealthy men with political power and influence. They would have to spend money on improvements. Many of them resented this. A few did not. Robert Owen set up a new mill in Lanarkshire. The workers had homes, fair wages and good surroundings. Owen found that they worked better. His profits rose. This change benefited all concerned. Source J shows the things that one of the local boards of health tried to do.

Source J. Effects of the local board of health.

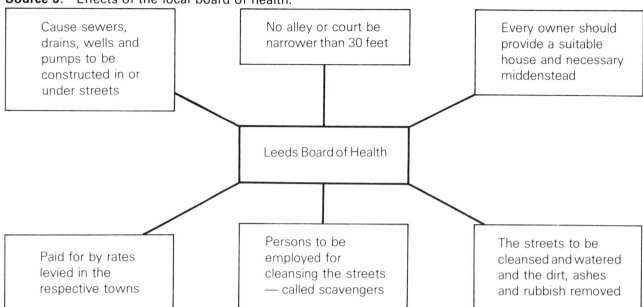

Cause sewers, drains, wells and pumps to be constructed in or under streets	No alley or court be narrower than 30 feet	Every owner should provide a suitable house and necessary middenstead
	Leeds Board of Health	
Paid for by rates levied in the respective towns	Persons to be employed for cleansing the streets — called scavengers	The streets to be cleansed and watered and the dirt, ashes and rubbish removed

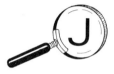

Public health had returned to Britain. It had not really existed there since the Roman Legions left.

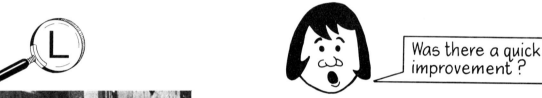

Was there a quick improvement?

No. It took a long time. It is still being improved. The Government passed the first Public Health Act in 1848. This did not do very much. A better Act was passed in 1875. Source K is from 'Medicine Through Time' (Holmes McDougall, 1987).

Source K

'From this time onwards all town councils were compelled to provide an adequate clean water supply, a proper system of drainage and sewage, and also appoint a Medical Officer of Health'.

There was still a lot of disease. Many babies died. Families were big but a lot of children died before they reached the age of five years. There was poverty and hunger. Source L shows people in London's East End getting food parcels. This was in the early 1900s.

Look at Source L
? Are these people rich or poor? How do you know?
? What do you notice about their clothes?
? Do they look clean? Why?
? Do they look as if they have plenty to eat?
? How might all these things affect their health?

The Government kept trying to improve things. The most important thing that the Government did was to start the National Health Service in 1947–8. Everyone in the country had the right to free medical treatment. Doctors and nurses were well trained. Hospitals were improved and anyone could go to them. Everyone had the right to modern treatments and sensible cures. Progress at last.

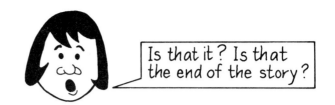

Is that it? Is that the end of the story?

No. Of course not. Doctors are still improving medicine. Scientists are discovering something new and useful every day. People live longer. They are much healthier. This century has seen some of the biggest advances in medicine. You have seen how the foundations for this were laid thousands of years ago.

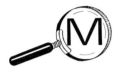

Source M shows important Acts that improved and changed medicine in this country. Copy the table in your book. Fill in the columns saying which people each Act helped. How do you think each Act improved life in the towns in Britain?

Act	Who it helped	How do you think each Act changed life for the people?
1. 1902 Midwives Act 1918 Midwives Act These Acts improved training for midwives. Midwives had to be registered with the government.		
2. 1907 Notification of Birth Act Each baby born had to be registered.		
3. 1918 Maternity and Child Welfare Act This Act provided benefits such as milk and hospital care for mothers and babies.		
4. 1906 Education and School Meals Act 1907 School Medical Service Act These Acts provided education for all children, cheap meals and regular medical inspections.		
5. 1911 National Health Insurance Act Every worker paid a small amount of money. If he was ill he got some payment.		
6. 1908 Old Age Pensions Act This gave a small amount of money every week to men and women over 65 years.		
7. 1909 Town Planning Act 1919 Housing Act 1930 Housing Act These Acts were to improve towns and houses. Sewage, drainage and water supplies were improved.		

What sort of discoveries or improvements in Public Health or medicine might be made in the future? Look around your locality. List all of the things that are done to improve public health in your area.

Medicine today and tomorrow

The final section of Unit 12 is for you to do some research.

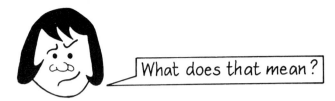

It means finding out things for yourself. You should consult books, magazines, newspapers, television, videos, radio and leaflets. Your teacher or your library or both will be able to help you.

Drugs

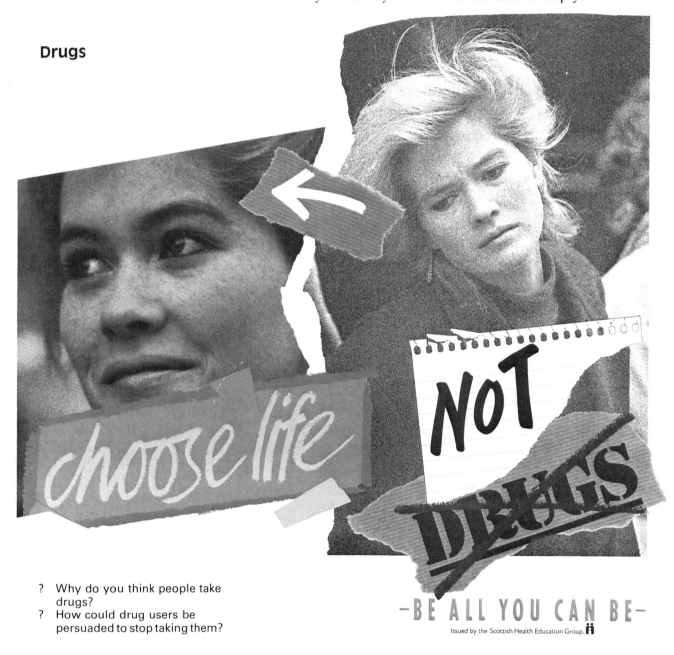

? Why do you think people take drugs?

? How could drug users be persuaded to stop taking them?

We hear about drugs nearly every day on television or at school. Gather as much information as you can about drugs. This might be notes from television programmes, leaflets from school or your local health centre, newspaper and magazine cuttings, and interviews. Make a scrap-book section about drugs in your book.

92

World health

We have heard a lot about disease and starvation. These problems still exist in many parts of the world today. Find out as much as you can about medical problems in the world today. You might research the following things:

(a) **Famine.** Which countries suffer from famine today? Why? What can other countries do to help?

(b) **Over feeding and heart disease.** Which countries are most likely to suffer from this problem? What can they do about it?

(c) **Traffic accidents.** Why are traffic accidents such a new problem?

(d) **Smoking.** Why do people smoke if it can kill them?

(e) **AIDS** and other diseases that cannot be cured, such as some kinds of cancer.

? Choose one world health problem and find out as much as you can about it. Write down how you think people could try to solve this problem.

? What do you know about AIDS? Do you think enough information about AIDS is given out on the TV and in newspapers?

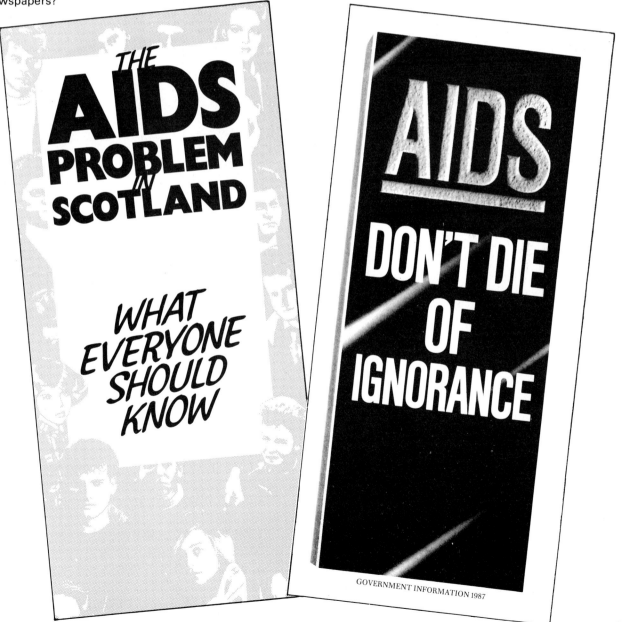

Alternative medicine

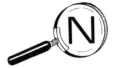

There is a big move towards fitness at the moment. Collect all the leaflets and advertisements that you can find that mention health and fitness.

People are becoming aware that drugs and chemicals are not the only answer to illness. Many people are returning to herbal medicine to give natural cures. Source N (a) and (b) show us that there is nothing new about herbal medicine. Many drugs are naturally produced by plants, such as aspirin.

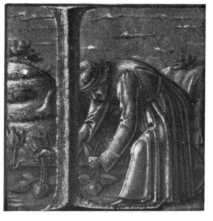

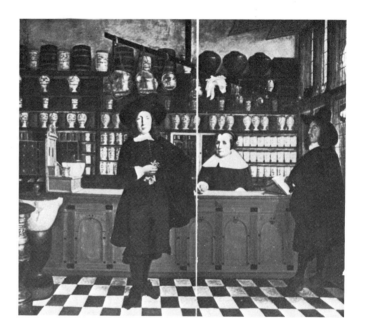

? List all the fitness ideas around today. Are there new ideas?
? Why do people use herbal medicine?
? Explain alternative medicine in your own words.

Many people now turn to better and natural foods with no additives. A lot of people visit osteopaths to cure physical problems. Some even use acupuncture. Is this idea new?

Maternity care

Fashions are changing in looking after mothers and new babies. Look at Source O. Try talking to two mothers who had their babies years apart. You could ask your grandma and your mum. Find out if they went to hospital or not. Ask them what sort of treatment they got. How were the new babies looked after? Try writing to the following people to get information:
(a) The local clinic or health centre.
(b) Any nurses or midwives.
(c) The local maternity hospital.
(d) The local branch of the National Childbirth Trust.

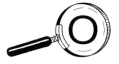

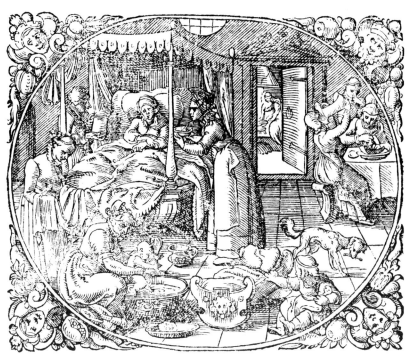

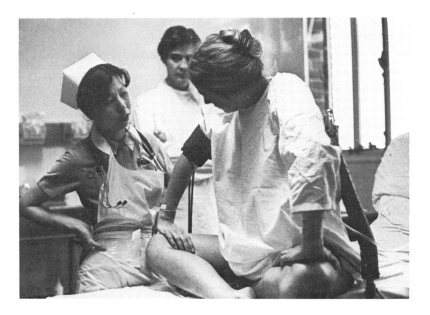

This section is for you to find out for yourself. Collect as much information as you can. It will all be useful to you. Medicine today is what keeps **you** well. Discover as much as you can.

We have seen the development of medicine over thousands of years. We have seen advances. We have seen steps backwards. The future remains to be seen.

Acknowledgements

The author and the publisher acknowledge the following illustration sources. They have made every effort to trace the copyright holders but where they have failed they will be happy to make the neccessary arrangements at the first opportunity.

We are grateful to the following for permission to reproduce illustrations:

Anthropological Institute, Florence **11, 23**
Australian Museum, Sydney **14**
BBC Hulton **16, 54, 66, 67, 70, 71, 72**
Geoffrey Berry **36**
Bodleian Library **94**
British Museum **18, 19, 20, 21**
Cambridge University Library **44**
Churchill Livingstone **89**
Department of Health and Social Security **93**
Edinburgh Royal Infirmary **4, 11, 83**
Mary Evans **22, 26, 82, 90**
Glasgow Art Gallery, Kelvingrove **47**
Frank Graham, Publisher/R. Embleton **38**
Her Majesty the Queen **58**
HMSO **37**
Herald & Weekly Times, Melbourne/Sir Balwin Spencer **13**
Howorth Air Conditioning **76**
Instituto Serono, Rome **27**
Leeds Public Library **87**
Liverpool Museums **29**
Mansell Collection **28, 29, 32, 33, 34, 55, 57, 69, 71, 79, 80, 81, 82, 83**
Douglas Mazonowicz, Gallery of Prehistoric Art **6**
National Childbirth Trust **95**
Oxfam **49**
Piraeus Museum **31**
Prähistorische Abteilung, Naturhistorisches Museum, Vienna **9**
Punch **73**
Ann Ronan **65, 74, 75**
Royal College of Physicians **60, 63, 89**
St. Bartholomew's Hospital **46**
Scottish Health Education Group **92, 93**
Sefton Photo Library **35**
J. S. Varley **86**
Wellcome Institute **27, 41, 50, 59, 61, 64, 65, 68, 70, 73, 84, 95**